BABY-LED WEANING

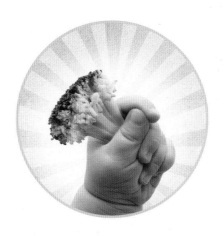

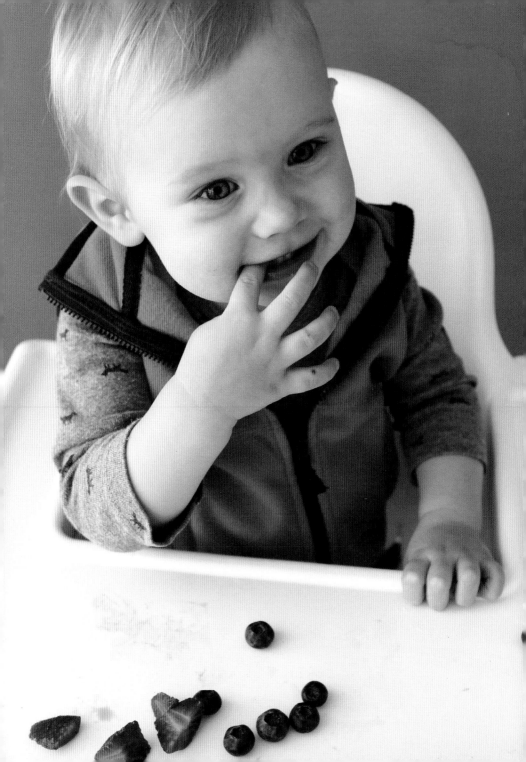

BABY-LED
WEANING

The (Not-So) Revolutionary Way
to Start Solids and Make a Happy Eater

Teresa Pitman

Foreword by Dr. Jack Newman

FIREFLY BOOKS

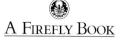

A FIREFLY BOOK

Published by Firefly Books Ltd. 2018
Copyright © 2018 Firefly Books Ltd.
Text copyright © Teresa Pitman 2018
Photographs © as listed on page 189

First printing

Library of Congress Control Number: 2018937296

Library and Archives Canada Cataloguing in Publication
Pitman, Teresa, author
      Baby-led weaning : the (not-so) revolutionary way to
start solids and make a happy eater / Teresa Pitman ; foreword
by Dr. Jack Newman, M.D.
Includes bibliographical references and index.
ISBN 978-0-228-10065-2 (softcover)
      1. Infants--Weaning. 2. Infants--Nutrition. I. Title.
RJ216.P58 2018   649'.3   C2018-901620-5

Published in the United States by
Firefly Books (U.S.) Inc.
P.O. Box 1338, Ellicott Station
Buffalo, New York 14205

Published in Canada by
Firefly Books Ltd.
50 Staples Avenue, Unit 1
Richmond Hill, Ontario L4B 0A7

Cover and interior design: Tania Craan

Printed in China

Canada We acknowledge the financial support of the Government of Canada.

Disclaimer: The nutritional, medical and health information presented in this book is based on the research of the author, and is true and complete to the best of her knowledge. This book is intended as an informative guide for those wanting to learn more about baby-led weaning and is not intended to substitute or challenge the advice given by the reader's pediatrician or a qualified medical professional. Because each baby and situation is unique, the author and publisher urge the reader to check with a qualified medical professional if the reader is unsure of the appropriateness of a particular course of action. The author and the publisher are not responsible for any loss, injury or damage that may arise from the use of the information in this book. It is the reader's responsibility to consult a qualified healthcare professional regarding his or her baby's personal care and well-being. The opinions expressed in this book represent the personal views of the author and not of the publisher.

For Julian and Kai,
my 9th and 10th grandchildren,
who arrived as we finished up this book.

Table of Contents

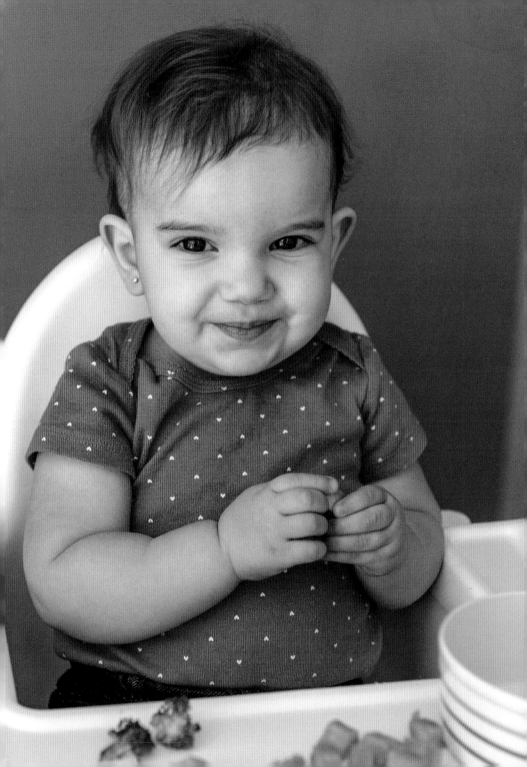

Foreword

Once upon a time, not so long ago, we didn't stress about giving food other than breast milk to babies. When babies were ready, they were given solid food, usually the same food their parents were eating.

The title of this book, *Baby-Led Weaning*, is actually a term that was coined in the UK. There, "weaning" means adding food to breastfeeding (while in North America, the word typically suggests the end of breastfeeding). These days, many view six months of breastfeeding as a milestone that, once reached, means that whatever happens with breastfeeding afterward is just fine, the mother's duty is done. It's not. One key message that this book wishes to get across is that six months is not the time to cut down on breastfeeding, to substitute food for breastfeeding or to stop breastfeeding at night or in accordance with the baby's needs. Rather, six months is the time to add food to undiminished breastfeeding and the beginning of many months when babies learn to eat food and enjoy different tastes and textures.

Recently, breastfeeding and starting foods have become riddled with dos and don'ts and so many rules that they make mothers fear breastfeeding even before giving birth and parents dread the time when their babies try their first foods. Instead of being enjoyed, these stages have become monumental academic projects in "how to get it right." Instead of feeling lucky to have food, people have begun worrying whether each piece in front of them contains the correct nutrition. In fact, we can say that people in much of the developed world no longer eat food, they eat nutrition.

As an example, formula is advertised as full of iron and vitamins and a necessity for a baby's health. "Follow-up" formula after the first six months and onward has become an even larger market than formula before the first six months, and its use has come to be stretched out beyond the age of one — well into toddlerhood — up to the ages of three and even five. This is a perfect example of eating nutrition instead of food. Why give children a variety of healthy foods when you can just give them a bland-tasting, processed drink of nutrition?

With this demand for formula comes an explosion of other processed, ready-to-eat baby foods: infant cereals, pureed vegetables, pouches with fruit (that are jam packed with sugar), combinations of formula and porridges — all with a taste that never changes. There is now a whole world of baby fast food out there, and formula and baby food companies are investing a lot of money to convince customers that these processed baby products are better and healthier than real food, not to mention more convenient — there's no need to peel a banana or even take a bite.

Like breastfeeding, starting a baby on the path to enjoying solid food should be much simpler than all those complicated tables and manuals suggest. Never have we worried about our children's food and nutrition more than at this point in history, when we, ironically, have the largest quantities of food available.

It is time to stop worrying, to stop creating rules and to allow babies to reach for food, put it in their mouths and eat just like everyone else in the family.

– Jack Newman, MD, FRCPC, IBCLC

Introduction

As a longtime La Leche League Leader, I've spent countless hours helping parents solve breastfeeding problems. Of course, breastfeeding isn't the only thing new parents want to talk about! Sleep (and the lack of it) is another major concern. And once they get through the first few months, many parents start wondering about the when and how of starting solid foods.

A generation or two ago, parents were generally advised to give solid foods very early. That meant spooning pureed foods into babies' mouths, since tiny babies can't handle anything else. But even back then research began to question this approach, finding fault with both early solids and the spoon-feeding method.

I've always followed and advocated La Leche League's advice to start offering solid foods around the middle of the first year and to provide finger foods so babies can feed themselves. Research suggests starting solids this way helps to protect babies against infections and reduces the risk of children later becoming obese or overweight. The baby-led approach reached a broader audience when, in 2008, a British nurse named Gill Rapley wrote the book *Baby-Led Weaning* and it hit bookstores worldwide.

The term "baby-led weaning" may be a bit confusing to North American readers because we generally use the word "weaning" to mean ending breastfeeding (or feeding with a bottle) completely. So, in this sense, baby-led weaning means allowing the baby to continue breastfeeding until she loses interest on her own. In the UK, though, weaning simply means starting solid foods. As the book and Rapley's approach became more popular, mommy blogs and parenting publications in North America started using the term as well. Some use "baby-led solids" so as not to confuse Rapley's expression with the North American meaning. However, we are using baby-led weaning here as it's the most popular term for this approach.

Research and terminology aside, my experience with baby-led weaning for my own children and grandchildren has been overwhelmingly positive. Look at the photos in this book and you'll see what I mean: babies and toddlers clearly enjoy being able to choose, pick up and tackle foods themselves. They're developing skills that will benefit them through a lifetime of eating, and they're learning to listen to their bodies about what and how much they need to eat.

I hope this book helps you as you plan to introduce your own baby to new foods. We've got lots of information for you here, including sections on starting solids if your family is vegan, vegetarian or paleo and some easy recipes your baby will love. But first we'll start with a little girl named Isla — who happens to be my granddaughter — and her experiences with baby-led weaning.

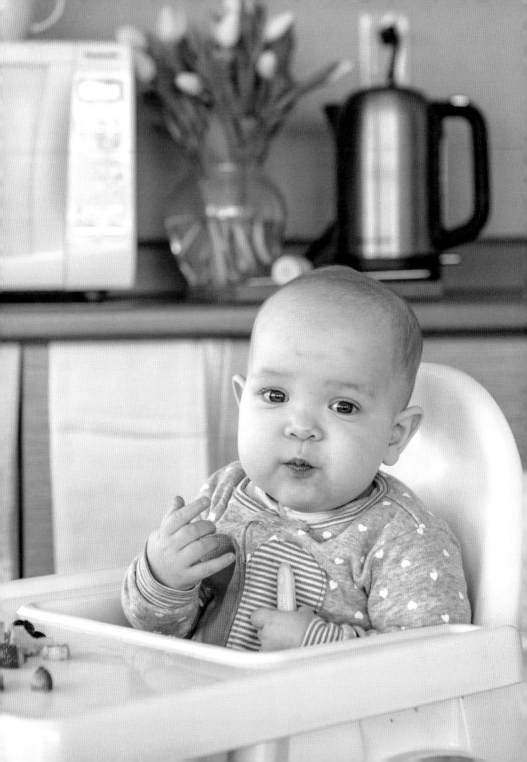

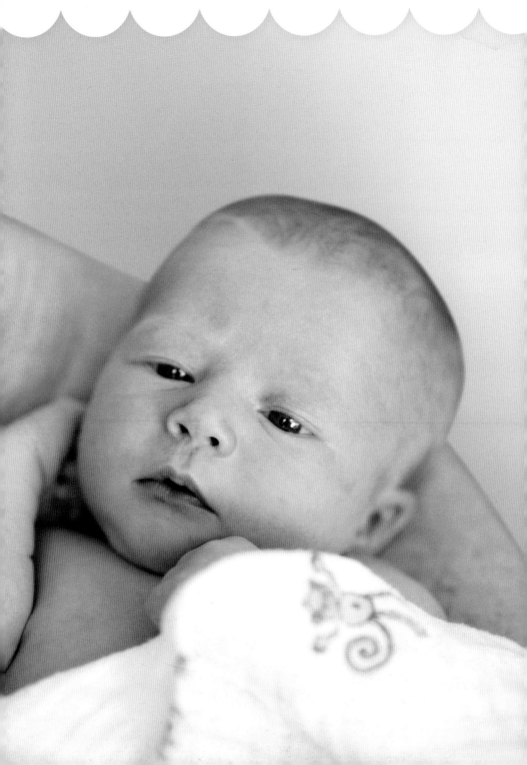

1

Isla's Journey to Eating Solids

Meet Isla. In this chapter you will join her and her parents, Lisa and Sascha, on a journey as she discovers solid foods and learns how to become a happy, healthy eater.

Isla was born on her due date at home in Toronto, Canada, weighing 8 pounds and 1 ounce (3.7 kg). At first, her mother, Lisa, was so relieved and delighted just to have her baby born that she didn't even check to see if she'd had a boy or girl as she snuggled her newborn against her chest. The midwife covered mother and baby with a blanket to keep them both warm, and it was only a few minutes later that Lisa asked, "Is it a boy or a girl?"

Lisa and her partner, Sascha, peeked under the blanket and got their answer: it was a girl. They named her Isla. Isla didn't have much hair at first, but as it began to grow in over the following weeks, they could see it was red, like her father's, and her eyes were blue.

Lisa had always planned to breastfeed, so she was delighted when Isla latched on and began to nurse within minutes of her birth.

⋙ Searching for Signs

Isla grew up fast on her mother's milk, and soon enough Lisa needed to start thinking about the next step: starting solid foods. She started reading a lot on the subject, and, as a vegan, she paid particular attention to information about healthy foods for vegan babies.

She knew that 6 months was the recommended age for starting solids and that parents should also watch for signs of readiness, but she wasn't quite sure what those were.

Like all babies, Isla couldn't do much at first. She relied on her parents to move her around. She could grab a finger if someone touched her palm, but she couldn't reach out to pick something up. She couldn't sit up at all, but she could recline in a bouncy seat or car seat. Within a few months, though, she was much more capable. By 3 months, she could reliably hold up her head and grab toys that were offered to her. She was also showing more and more interest in the world around her, which included watching her parents eat.

Isla's feeding behaviors were changing, too. When she was almost 4 months old, she went through a couple of days of very frequent nursing. Lisa had come to count on Isla having a couple of hours between feedings most of the time, but suddenly she was back to nursing like a newborn. Had Lisa's milk supply dropped? Was Isla sick? Or was this a sign that Isla was ready to eat solid foods? Sure, she was only 4 months old, but some babies start a bit early, right?

Lisa got in touch with a La Leche League Leader to see whether this was normal and what she could do if it wasn't. La Leche League is an international organization of experienced breastfeeding mothers who take some additional training to prepare them for providing support and information to other breastfeeding women. Lisa learned that many babies go through a growth spurt at this age and nurse more frequently for a few days to increase milk production. As the Leader predicted, Isla settled back into her previous pattern after a few days.

The next change Lisa noticed at around 4 months was that Isla was much more distractible. As a young baby, Isla was totally focused on breastfeeding when she was at the breast. A herd of wild horses followed by a fleet of ambulances wouldn't have distracted her from nursing; all she cared about was getting that milk. But when Isla was around 4 months, Lisa found it increasingly frustrating to nurse her anywhere but in a quiet room. Even the sound of people talking outside their apartment would cause Isla to drop the nipple and turn her head away from the breast to see what was going on. Even worse, Isla sometimes didn't let go of the nipple before turning her head to look around!

In Canada, visit www.lllc.ca to find a local La Leche League Leader or group.

In the U.S. and other countries, visit www.llli.org. The site will refer you to your country's La Leche League website, where you can find information about local Leaders and groups.

Sometimes Isla would stop several times during a feeding just to check out the world. Even while she was actually suckling, she'd fiddle with her clothing or twist strands of Lisa's long hair in her hand or poke her fingers in Lisa's mouth. (Parents of babies this age sometimes joke that they get a free dental exam with every feeding.)

Was this a sign that Isla was losing interest in nursing? Was she ready for solid foods?

There was another behavior that made Lisa wonder. At 4 and 5 months, Isla often sat on her mother's or father's laps while they were eating. Sascha, her father, noticed that she seemed quite interested in the food on his plate, and sometimes when he moved a green bean or a forkful of mashed potatoes to his mouth, she'd watch him carefully and get excited. Sometimes she'd reach her hands out toward the plate and poke her fingers into the food.

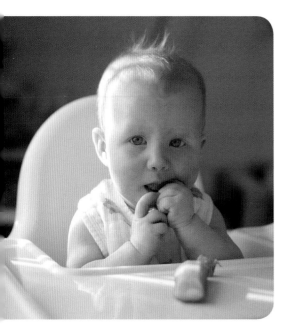

Isla often picked up toys and put them in her mouth, but Lisa noticed that Isla didn't really seem to want to eat them. Instead, she seemed to be using this as another way to explore the world: what does this taste like? How does it feel in my mouth?

Lisa and Sascha had already decided that they wanted to try the baby-led weaning approach to starting solid foods, but they wondered how they'd know when it was time to start offering solid food to Isla.

A La Leche League Leader provided Lisa with these guidelines for readiness:

1. Isla is able to sit up comfortably without support. This makes it possible for her to pick up food, put it in her mouth and be in control of the process.

2. Isla has the dexterity needed to pick up objects and move them to her mouth.

3. Isla no longer has the "tongue extrusion reflex" seen in younger babies. Young babies will automatically use their tongues to push solid foods (or other things) back out of their mouths. To eat solids, she needs to be able to move the food from the front of her mouth to the back, where it is swallowed.

4. Isla shows interest in food, perhaps reaching for food from Sascha's plate or watching intently as Lisa eats.

All four of these signs need to be in place before Isla starts solid foods.

⊳→ Isla's First Foods

Isla was just around her 6-month birthday when Lisa decided to give solids a try. She had been watching with interest when her parents ate, and the other physical abilities detailed by the La Leche League guidelines were present. It felt like a big step to Lisa, but Isla seemed ready.

With Isla sitting on her lap at the table, Lisa put some cubes of baked sweet potato on a plastic mat in front of her. Before serving it to Isla, Lisa had removed the peel and let the sweet potato cool to room temperature. Sweet potato is often a good choice for a baby's first food — the bright color

Isla's Evolution

Lisa and Sascha took Isla's photo every month for her first year. You can see how Isla has grown from a newborn with very little hand control to a confident toddler with great self-feeding skills who knows what foods she likes and dislikes.

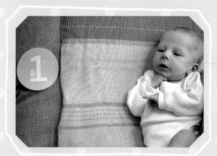

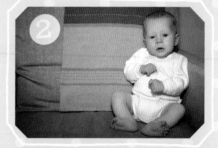

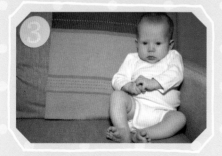

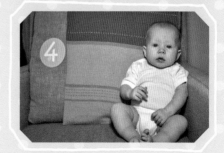

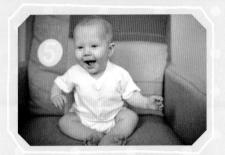

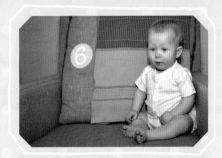

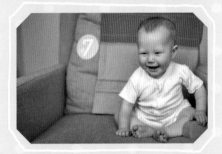

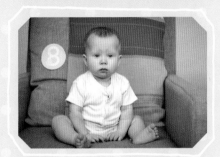

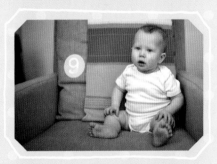

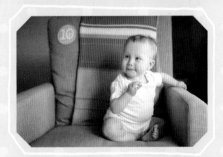

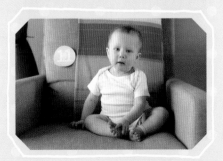

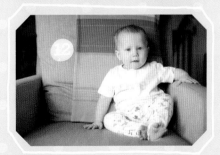

attracts a baby's interest, it's soft enough when cooked for most babies to manage easily and the mild, slightly sweet taste is likely to appeal to a baby.

It certainly appealed to Isla! She scooped up a cube, squished it a bit with her hand and popped it into her mouth. She moved it around her mouth, mushed it up, swallowed it and then reached out for more.

This first time Isla ate only three pieces, but Lisa was delighted that it had gone so well.

Starting One Food at a Time

Because Lisa comes from a family with quite a few allergies, she was careful to offer just one food at a time in the beginning. The reason for doing this was simple: if Isla had an allergic reaction, Lisa could readily identify the cause.

At first, Isla ate solids just once a day; the rest of the time she breastfed as usual. After a couple of weeks of one food once a day, Lisa started offering solids twice daily and including more than one food with each meal, which she selected from the foods she and Sascha were eating for their meals. She bought a plate that was divided into sections to keep the foods separate. She also bought a high chair that allowed Isla to eat at the table beside her parents.

By 8 months, Isla was eating three meals a day with her parents, as well as nursing frequently. This won't be true of all babies. At this stage, some may eat only a few pieces of solid food each day and continue relying mostly on breast milk or formula for their nutrition. That's fine, too.

Letting Isla Choose

At every meal, Isla would get a little buffet spread of food options on her plate. Lisa wanted her to be able to choose what appealed to her on that particular day. Lisa gradually increased the quantity of each food and provided more choices at each meal. She made a point of naming each food as she put it on Isla's plate so that Isla would know what the foods were called.

As Isla got older, Lisa began combining more foods. She would mix together something Isla already liked with something new — mashing some sweet potato with cooked lentils, for example, or making whole-grain muffins with blueberries. Pieces of pita stuffed with food and crepes wrapped around tasty fillings were popular options with Isla.

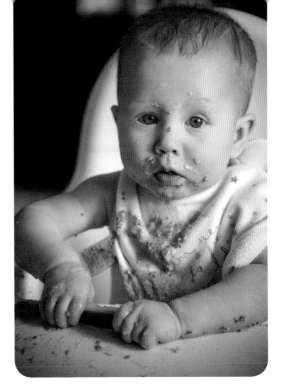

Sometimes Isla would reject one of the foods Lisa offered. Bananas are favorites for many babies, but the first time Lisa put a "finger" of banana on Isla's plate, her daughter looked at it with suspicion. After eating a few other things, Isla put the banana in her mouth briefly and then put it back down. Lisa tried banana again a few days later and Isla pushed it to the side. It took several more tries before Isla was willing to taste it again, and she took a couple of small bites. Maybe, she seemed to decide, this strange, whitish fruit wasn't so bad after all.

Like most of us, Isla's appetite fluctuated from meal to meal and day to day. Sometimes she'd eat a lot, sometimes just a little. When Isla had had enough, she'd let her parents know by pushing the food away or trying to get out of her high chair. It was tempting at times to encourage her to eat the last few peas or blueberries, but Lisa tried to respect that Isla was listening to her body's messages about how much food she needed.

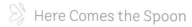

Early on, Isla was interested in the utensils her parents were using and sometimes grabbed for a knife or spoon. When Isla was 10 months old, Lisa bought her a small wooden spoon with a fairly thick handle. Lisa would put a little food on it — maybe a thick soup that she was having with her lunch — and put it down for Isla to try. Often, most of the food fell off as Isla tried to get the spoon into her mouth, but usually enough clung to the spoon that Isla was able to get a taste.

Soon, Isla was using the spoon to scoop up yogurt or hummus, though not very effectively. She had better luck with pieces of pita bread or fairly firm vegetables. It wasn't until she passed 16 months that she could use the spoon effectively enough to transfer food to her mouth.

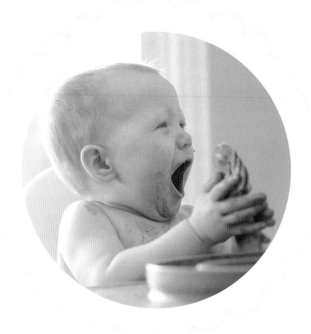

⤳ Carrying On

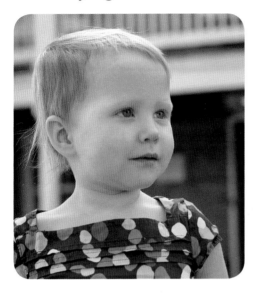

At 22 months, Isla is still making her own food choices, and because her mother names all the foods she serves, Isla can identify a wide range of foods. On trips to the grocery store, she'll happily point out clementines, mangoes, brussels sprouts and other favorites, and she can now request the foods she wants her mother to prepare. She's also able to eat more things combined into casseroles or wraps, now that her parents know which foods she's allergic to and which foods are safe. Lisa still breastfeeds several times a day and at night, and she doesn't see that ending anytime soon.

For Isla's second birthday — which is coming up — she's already told her mother she wants crepes to be served and for all her friends and family to attend.

Lisa feels good about how baby-led weaning has worked out for Isla, who has learned to enjoy healthy foods and to listen to her body about how much to eat. Lisa's goal is to continue this pattern and create a solid foundation for Isla's future.

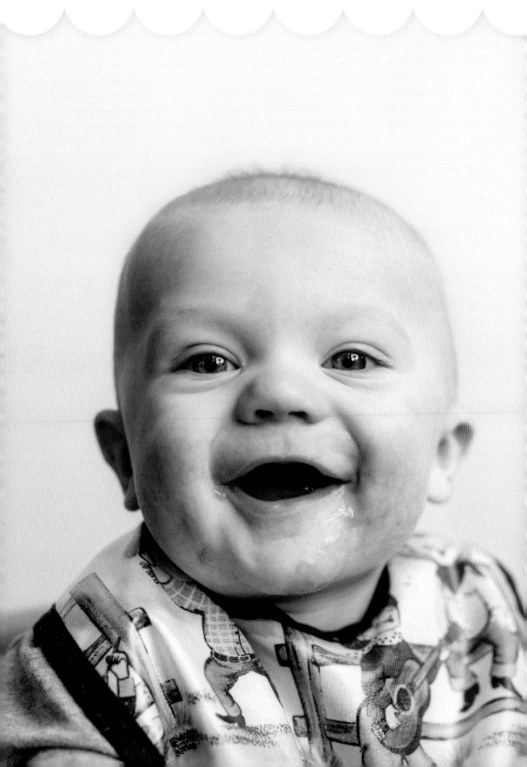

2

A History of Feeding Babies

Those processed infant cereals and jars or pouches of baby food are all recent inventions. Knowing a little about the history of infant feeding can put this in perspective and help you understand what — and how — babies have evolved to eat. This chapter will also help you understand where your baby's grandparents are coming from if they criticize the baby-led approach to starting solids.

Sally: My mom was horrified when I told her that I was planning to wait until Nell was 6 months old to start offering her solid foods. She started me at 3 months, and she told me her mom — my grandma — had given her cereal by 6 weeks. There was just no way Nell could survive and get the nutrition she needed on just my milk for 6 months.

The past few generations of parents were advised to start solid foods within the first 6 months of a baby's life, and that means your baby's grandparents may be passing on that information to you, urging you to start adding solid foods to your baby's diet from very early on. Baby-led weaning might seem like some kind of dangerous new fad to parents from previous generations, and with the existence of so many foods designed for very young infants, today's supermarkets only seem to reaffirm their views.

Check the baby aisle in any grocery store and you will see: right next to the cans of formula and bottles of baby shampoo sit boxes of special cereals for infants, packaged teething biscuits and jars of pureed fruits, vegetables and "baby meals" like beef stew and spaghetti and meatballs. Next to them, you'll spot one of the newest approaches to feeding infants: pouches with fruit and vegetable purees that the baby can suck right out of the pouch.

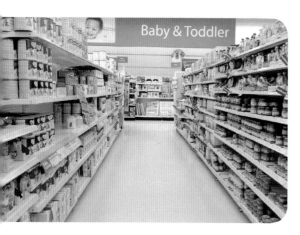

You also might see little mesh pouches with handles on them, another new strategy for giving infants solid foods. The idea is that a parent fills the pouch with pureed food and the baby sucks the puree through the mesh.

Looking at the all the food selections, many of which are processed so that young infants can swallow them, it's easy to think that all of these items are necessary for good nutrition for your growing baby. But what if they're not?

Have you ever wondered how babies started on solid foods before the creation of spoons, baby cereals, commercial baby foods and blenders? What did mothers feed their babies a few hundred years ago, when did they start their babies on solids and what can we learn from them? Or from other mammals?

Let's start with our mammal cousins.

⥸→ Mammal Babies

The word "mammal" comes from the Latin word for breast, *mamma*. Lactation is the defining factor for this family of animals, which we also belong to: all mammal babies start off drinking milk from their mothers' bodies. The composition of the milk varies from one species to another: some milks are higher in fat and protein, some are higher in milk sugar, but each meets the developmental needs and way of life of a particular species. For example, cows make milk that is high in protein, because a baby calf is already standing and walking within an hour or two of its birth and needs to continue developing strong muscles. Baby bats need to be left alone in a cave for hours at a time, while their mothers hunt mosquitoes and other bugs, so the milk they are fed is concentrated with lots of slow-digesting fats, which means they won't get hungry while mom is away. Gorilla milk, like human milk, is less concentrated and lower in both fat and protein because gorilla babies typically spend their days and nights in their mothers' arms, feeding

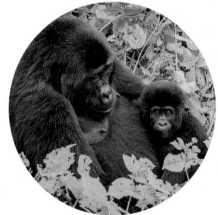

frequently around the clock. It also contains more components that are important for brain development, something essential for primates.

Over time, though, a growing baby begins to need other foods. By about 6 months, baby gorillas start imitating their mothers by putting leaves and pieces of fruit in their mouths, and by 8 months, they are usually eating a variety of typical gorilla foods. (You might be surprised to know that gorillas are vegan!) The mother does little to encourage or discourage this natural behavior, but since the baby is always in close contact with its mother, it has plenty of opportunities to see what and how she eats. And even though the little gorilla is eating other foods, it continues to nurse and drink its mother's milk for at least two years.

If you've ever owned a dog that has had puppies, you know that the process is considerably streamlined in the canine family. Puppies usually start eating solid foods at 3 or 4 weeks and may be completely weaned by 8 weeks (sometimes earlier if the owner is selling the puppies, or later if they are allowed to wean on their own). Puppies are quite eager to chew on anything their mouths come in contact with, chomping down on toys, shoes and people's fingers if they happen to grab them. So when they get a chance to try out the food in mama's bowl, that chewing instinct comes to the fore.

Human babies are much more like gorillas than puppies. We require that longer timeline for enjoying mother's milk before starting solids. This makes sense because, after all, we are primates, too.

ᗧ→ Baby Food Through the Ages

Thanks to the work of countless anthropologists, we know that before written history, human babies were fed pretty much the same way as the babies of other mammals — first with their mothers' milk and then sharing family foods as they grew. Some of those foods might have been cooked, others served raw. The parents might have chewed up some foods to make them soft enough to offer to the baby. This is still practiced in various communities in Africa and South America, and among some indigenous peoples in Canada, Australia and other countries who follow handed-down traditions. (Some experts warn against this for today's parents because cavity-causing bacteria can be transferred from the parent's mouth to the baby's mouth.) What about those situations when a breastfeeding mother didn't have enough milk or for other reasons wasn't able to provide all the milk her baby needed? That happened in the past just as it does today. In a given village or community, there would usually be another mother who could share her milk with a hungry baby, since most mothers can make more milk than one baby requires.

Over 3,000 years ago, right up until the 19th century, wealthier women sometimes hired "wet nurses" — women who cared for and breastfed their employers' babies. At times, women who couldn't afford wet nurses but needed to be away from their children or wanted to supplement their milk fed their babies with animal milks or a mixture of flour or cooked grains with water or animal milks (or other solid foods, depending on the time period and location), typically delivered in unsanitary feeding vessels. Unfortunately, a significant number of these babies died. In 1799, Dr. Michael Underwood wrote that in London, England, only one in eight non-breastfed babies survived.

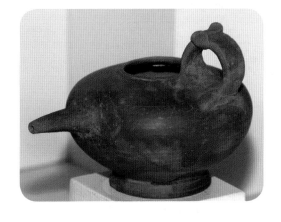

If a baby was still getting primarily human milk, her chances of survival improved, but otherwise she was at risk in two ways: one, the food she was fed was unlikely to have all the nutrients she needed to survive; two, these concoctions lacked the antibodies and immune factors found in breast milk that would protect her from disease.

Formula

Because each mammal makes milk specific to the needs of its species, early attempts to feed human babies with milk from other mammals were not very successful, and the babies often became ill or died. Doctors realized early on that the milks obtained from domesticated animals, such as cows and goats, would need to be modified in some way to make them more closely resemble human milk. In particular, these doctors needed to decrease the level of protein and increase the sugar.

Homemade Formulas • The earliest formulas were devised in the 1800s and were literally based on sets of instructions, like chemistry formulas. The doctor would write a step-by-step method for the parents to mix up a formula for the baby: pour in a certain amount of cow's milk, add a certain amount of sugar and water, heat and feed. As the baby grew, the proportions could be adjusted. After 1856, when Eagle Brand founder Gail Borden patented the process of condensing milk in a vacuum, sweetened condensed milk was sometimes recommended as the base for the formula. Canned milk was safer than fresh milk because refrigeration hadn't yet been invented; a formula-fed baby lacked the antibodies and anti-infective components he would have gotten from human milk, so he was very susceptible to any bacteria that might grow in milk.

Formula recipes continued to be prescribed for new babies well into the 1960s and, in certain areas, beyond that time. In fact, homemade formulas remain popular in some communities in Atlantic Canada today.

Of course, these homemade formulas were deficient in a number of ways: they were susceptible to contamination with bacteria, and tired parents could make errors in mixing up the ingredients from time to time. A 2013 study by de Carvalho and Morais found that the calorie, protein and carbohydrate levels were higher than recommended in 75 percent of the homemade formulas that were tested, and almost all were contaminated with bacteria.

Commercial Formulas • The first commercial formula was created by Justus von Liebig in 1865 and was made with cow's milk, wheat flour, malt flour and potassium bicarbonate. (Doesn't sound very tasty, does it?) In 1867, Swiss entrepreneur Henri Nestle saw a way to improve von Liebig's formulation, and he mixed crumbs of wheat rusk with sweetened condensed milk to make "Nestle's milk food" for babies. He promoted this as being better for babies than human milk. (Spoiler: it was not.)

Schedules • Many parents saw these formulas — which were enthusiastically marketed, first to doctors and then to the public — as convenient, and they fit well into the new approaches to baby care recommended by some of the leading pediatricians of the time, such as Dr. John Watson, who published his very popular book *Psychological Care of Infant and Child* in 1928. Dr. Watson favored a very rigid approach to caring for infants. Babies were supposed to be kept on strict schedules for feeding, and cuddling was generally forbidden. Dr. Watson did permit parents to kiss the baby on the forehead — but just once a day. Rules that limited feeding and contact were much easier for the formula-feeding parent to follow.

Why would it be harder for a breastfeeding parent to follow this kind of schedule? First, because breastfeeding works best for most parents and babies when the baby's feeding cues are responded to. The baby adjusts both the quantity and composition of the milk by feeding more or less frequently and changing the length of time she spends at the breast. For example, frequent feedings, especially in the early

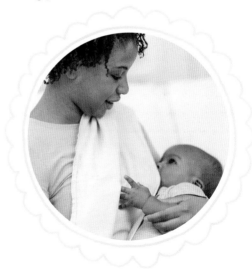

weeks of her life, promote the establishment of a good milk supply in her mother's body. Frequent feedings also increase the fat content in the milk, and frequent but short feedings give the baby more liquid, which is ideal for hotter weather. Feeding according to a schedule disrupts this natural process and can cause a reduction in a mother's milk supply.

Second, mothers vary considerably in their milk storage capacity. If a mother has a large storage capacity in her breasts, she can give her baby more at each feeding and then go longer between feedings. If she has a smaller storage capacity, she'll need to feed her baby more often — although she can produce the same amount of milk in total for her baby. So the three- or four-hour schedules recommended by Dr. Watson and his followers could work for a small percentage of nursing mothers, but would create serious problems for others.

Third, breastfeeding mothers find it much harder to follow a schedule because they can't bear hearing their babies cry. Research done at Yale University by James Swain and his colleagues showed that when breastfeeding mothers hear their babies cry, their brains react in the areas associated with nurturing and where "obsessive" behavior originates. In other words, when mothers hear their babies cry, their brains tell them to respond to their babies — and to be obsessive about it! This doesn't mesh well with the restrictions of scheduled feedings.

Finally, breastfeeding mothers have another physical response to the sound of their babies' cries: their milk will "let down" and can make their breasts feel uncomfortably full. The natural response is to breastfeed — not just to calm the baby, but to relieve their own discomfort. (Of course, a nursing mother typically wouldn't wait until her baby is crying. Crying is considered a late signal of hunger, and parents are encouraged to watch for the early signs, such as squirming, searching for the breast, sucking on hands or fingers and so on.)

With the increasing interest in formula use during the 20th century, more manufacturers stepped up and began selling ready-mixed substitutes for human milk. Formula was marketed as more scientific and reliable, something that won people over during those years of rapid scientific and medical advancements.

But even the new and improved formulas were problematic. Doctors continued to be concerned about the evidence of health and developmental problems based on research and their own observations.

One solution was attempted in Toronto, Canada. In 1931, three doctors from the Hospital for Sick Children, Dr. Frederick Tisdall, Dr. Theodore Drake and Dr. Alan Brown, along with nutrition lab technician Ruth Herbert, became concerned about the cases of malnutrition in the formula-fed babies they were seeing in the hospital. They decided to create a solid food that could be given to quite young babies to help fill in the nutritional gaps. The cereal — named Pablum, after *pabulum*, the Latin word for food — was made of fully cooked ingredients that were then dried, ground and packaged so that busy parents only needed to add hot water to reconstitute the cereal.

This original Pablum was made with whole wheat, oatmeal, corn-meal, bone meal, Brewer's yeast and alfalfa, making it a source of several important vitamins and minerals. The doctors also added iron. The iron was important because cow's milk, unless heat-treated to break down some

All gone!

There are hundreds of mothers who could tell you to this day when and where it was that someone uttered the words Nestlé's Milk. Perhaps it was the Doctor—perhaps the nurse, perhaps some other mother. But what a change it did make! Baby seemed to pick up right away—never looked back again! Nestlé's Milk is good rich farm milk—every drop of the cream in it and every one of the vitamins. But it has been so treated that the most delicate baby can digest it and get all the goodness from it.

NESTLÉ'S MILK

NESTLÉ'S MILK FOOD—When baby has been well built up by Nestlé's Milk you won't be left wondering what to do next. Nestlé's Milk Food—for bigger babies—will carry the good work on. A card to Nestlé's, Department I.W., 6-d. Eastcheap, E.C.3, will bring you full particulars of Nestlé's Milk Food.

components (as is done in modern commercial formulas), causes intestinal bleeding in young infants, which can lead to anemia. In the 1930s, most families were still making formulas at home, and many offered plain cow's milk at an early age, so this was a concern.

This original Pablum is quite different from the cereals currently marketed for infants, which are usually made of highly processed grains that have the fiber and other components removed and some vitamins and minerals added back in.

⊳→ The Myth of the Early Start

Ann: When I had my first baby in 1977, most new mothers stayed in the hospital for five days. I had a roommate whose baby was two days older than mine. When her son was 5 days old, her doctor told her to start giving him cereal. I remember sitting up in my bed, holding my newborn baby and watching my roommate spoon cereal into her 5-day-old baby's mouth. That seemed crazy early to me, but it was her doctor's standard advice.

By the early to mid-1940s, doctors were recommending that formula-feeding parents should be adding solid foods earlier and earlier. (In time, they began to recommend this to breastfeeding parents as well, though there was no evidence to support this advice.) After the end of World War II, 6 weeks had become the standard age, and that advice continued for several decades. However, some doctors encouraged parents to start even earlier, sometimes within a week of the baby being born.

Parents often didn't need a lot of encouragement — many saw starting solids as a developmental milestone. It also was seen as helpful if the mother was breastfeeding, because she could take a break from the baby if she wanted to without having to provide bottles.

Since doctors were recommending solid foods at such an early age, babies inevitably had to be spoon-fed; they simply didn't have the ability to self-feed. This ultimately created a whole industry of baby foods, because even soft, cooked foods mashed up by the parents might be too chunky for a 6-week-old (or younger!) baby to swallow easily. Some parents made home-made baby foods using blenders, but most purchased small jars of pureed foods, from single fruits to entire "dinners" that included meats, starches and vegetables.

Another popular strategy was to add cereal to a bottle of formula, enlarging the hole in the nipple so that the baby could just suck it out of the bottle. This increased the risk of overfeeding, as the cereal-thickened milk could just flow into the baby's mouth and he'd have to swallow so as not to choke.

Times have changed, and these are *not* the recommended practices today. But knowing about the enthusiasm the medical profession had for very early solids just a generation ago may help you to understand why your baby's grandparents might find baby-led weaning surprising — even worrisome. If they were told early solids were vital, how can it be safe to wait for six months, or even longer? And if they used a spoon and pureed food at the start, letting the baby pick up food and gnaw on it can seem dangerous.

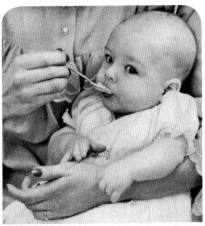

What makes baby's appetite g-r-o-w ?

At first, your cherub's hunger just naturally grows! But it's surprising how a healthy appetite can lag – unless Mommy takes a hand to keep baby really *interested* in eating.

You see, by the time your baby starts on strained foods, he also starts to de-

velop a greater sense of color and taste. So you'll notice that the more different varieties of Gerber's Strained Foods you give him, the more his appetite perks up. For Gerber's make a really *complete* choice for your little one's meal-times. And Gerber's take extra-special care to keep the tempting, natural color of each and every food . . . and the appetizing, individual true flavor, too!

Remember that Gerber's are also famous for the smooth-as-smooth texture that your baby enjoys . . . the wholesome goodness that you and your doctor look for.

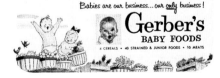

Babies are our business... our only business!

Gerber's
BABY FOODS
4 CEREALS • 40 STRAINED & JUNIOR FOODS • 10 MEATS

Blue-Ribbon Babies

The mid-1900s was also a time when the chubby baby was seen as ideal. Every mother wanted a "blue-ribbon" baby, and solid foods could be used to fatten up the baby who wasn't plump enough. Some mothers were even given booklets recommending fudge as the ideal food to fatten up a skinny baby. But too-rapid weight gain in infancy has since been linked to childhood and adult obesity, a significant problem in North America, where nearly one-third of adults are obese and the associated health problems are becoming an epidemic.

It's important to note that some breastfed babies do gain weight quickly in the first few months and can become very chubby. This normally resolves itself once the baby becomes mobile, in the second half of the first year, and the baby typically develops to a normal weight as a toddler. This is not the same situation as the baby who has been overfed on other foods.

The Risks of Early Solids for Breastfed Babies

These recommendations for introducing infant cereal and other foods early in life were not supported by research. Although many physicians were encouraging solids in the first couple of months after birth, research continued to indicate that starting solids later was associated with healthier babies and children, especially if the babies were breastfed.

To confirm this, the World Health Organization (WHO) reviewed the research and conducted its own studies involving thousands of babies from around the world. In 2003, the WHO issued a report entitled *Complementary Feeding: Report of the Global Consultation* that recommended exclusive breastfeeding from birth, introducing solids at around 6 months and continuing breastfeeding for two years and beyond. Why does the WHO advise waiting for six months to start offering solid foods? Because there are some real risks to adding foods other than human milk to a baby's diet too early.

Infections and Diseases • You probably know that exclusive breastfeeding reduces a baby's risk of catching various infections and diseases, including gastrointestinal illnesses (such as diarrheal disease), respiratory illnesses (such as influenza and pneumonia) and other illnesses (such as meningitis and ear infections). How does human milk do this? It contains several protective mechanisms.

One such mechanism is the secretory immunoglobulin A antibody. It coats the lining of the baby's entire digestive tract and helps to prevent bacteria and other microbes from getting into the baby's system and causing an infection. It even gets into the baby's nose at times when he sneezes milk or spits up — again, preventing bacteria from getting into his system through that avenue.

While keeping out the bad bacteria, human milk also provides food for the good bacteria. All of us have some good bacteria in our intestines that help us digest food, among other things. (The bacteria found in the intestinal tract are collectively known as gut flora.) We have learned in recent years that these bacteria play much more complex roles in our lives. For example, they influence our food choices, the development of our immune systems when we're babies and the expression of our genes. The types of bacteria present depend on our diet and other factors — taking antibiotics can wipe out a large number of the health-promoting good bacteria, for example. Breastfed babies have more of the protective bacteria than those fed formula, and these good bacteria fight any bad bacteria that get into the system and potentially cause disease.

When solid foods are added to a breastfed baby's diet, the bacterial balance in the baby's gut is disrupted. That makes the baby more vulnerable to infections, which can have serious consequences in some cases, especially when the baby is too young to have his own strong immune system. In fact, the WHO research showed that babies who started solids earlier had more infections. Even a mild infection can mean that the baby gets treated with antibiotics, which causes more changes to the baby's gut flora and leads to higher risks of health problems later. For example, a 2017 study led by Dr. Rebecca Slykerman found that being given antibiotics in infancy increased a person's risk of depression and behavioral problems in child-hood (ages 7 to 11 years). In 2016, research studies in the UK, the U.S. and Finland all pointed to increased weight gain among children who had been given antibiotics in infancy. (Farmers who raise animals for meat, such as chickens, cows and pigs, have long known that antibiotic use increases the rate of weight gain.)

So maintaining a baby on human milk as long as possible is important not only for that baby's immediate health, but also for his future health. As the baby gets older, his own immune system will start ramping up, and after 6 months or so, the negative effects of solid foods are less significant.

Human Milk Production • Starting solids too early can also displace human milk. Why does this matter? Every mammal species has a normal duration of lactation. For some, like dogs, it's measured in weeks. For primates — and humans are primates — the normal duration is usually two or more years. Research by anthropologist Kathy Dettwyler suggests that the normal age for ending breastfeeding in humans is between 30 months and 7 years.

But a lactating mother's ability to produce milk depends on that milk being removed from her body on a regular basis, and she is more sensitive to a decrease in milk removal when the baby is younger. If a baby starts solids at 3 months and is fed a significant amount of solid food, then the baby will be taking less breast milk and the mother's milk supply is likely to decrease. As this continues, it can lead to breastfeeding ending too early — and the baby misses out on the important antibodies and nutrition that continued breastfeeding would have provided.

Obesity • Finally, too-early solids are linked to excess weight and obesity. When babies are spoon-fed, it's easy for a parent to give the baby more than he wants. If the food is fairly liquid, such as a puree, it can trigger the swallowing reflex once it's in the baby's mouth, even if he really would rather spit it out. Parents also have a natural tendency to want to finish up the food in the bowl: if the baby seems uninterested but there is just a spoonful or two left, parents may want to spoon in those last bits of cereal or sweet potato. For a small baby, though, that extra food can be setting a lifelong pattern of eating beyond when he feels full.

So waiting until the baby is ready for solid foods, usually at around 6 months, has many important benefits.

⊳→ Baby-Led Weaning

While there are still a significant number of parents who are starting solids earlier than at 6 months, this is not what medical professionals recommend today. The WHO, Canadian Paediatric Society, American Academy of Pediatrics and others all consistently advise parents to wait until 6 months to introduce solid foods to their babies.

However, all those prepared cereals and pureed foods — which we now know were designed for less developed babies — are still filling up the store shelves, so parents often think that's what they should be using, especially if their ideas about infant feeding are being guided by information from their parents.

A new mother is advised by her doctor to start her baby on solid foods at 6 months. Her own mother talks about giving the baby infant cereal as a first food, and, sure enough, when this first-time mom checks the store, she sees boxes of processed cereal ready to be mixed into a smooth puree. Nearby are jars of pureed fruits, vegetables and meats. But when this mother brings the baby food home to her 6-month-old, she finds the feeding process does not go as smoothly as she anticipated. She tries to spoon some pureed food into her baby's mouth, but her baby grabs for the spoon. When the mother pulls the spoon away, the baby sticks both hands into the bowl and tries to feed herself. This 6-month-old baby is looking for a different approach to feeding than a 6-week-old baby, who cannot even hold his head up.

In 2008, British nurse Gill Rapley (alongside journalist Tracey Murkett) published a book called *Baby-Led Weaning*, coining the widely used term for this approach in the process. In the book, Rapley outlines the approach she has been suggesting to parents: letting the baby decide when to start eating solid foods and allowing the baby to self-feed. The book was met with considerable enthusiasm by many parents, and groups to support families using this approach started up around the world.

It's worth mentioning that La Leche League has been giving advice consistent with a baby-led approach since it was founded in 1956. This organization, created to support breastfeeding parents, has always recommended that solid foods begin around the middle of the first year, when a baby shows signs of readiness. The handouts and books produced by La Leche League to help mothers suggested 60 years ago — and still recommend today — that most babies by 6 months would be happier with finger foods the family enjoys than with purees or prepared infant cereals. Most parents involved with La Leche League have used a baby-led approach.

Despite the research and the recommendations, we're not quite there yet. A 2013 survey conducted by the Centers for Disease Control and Prevention in the U.S. found that about 40 percent of American parents start their babies on solid foods before 4 months. Nine percent start as early as 4 weeks. That's almost one in 10 babies getting solid foods in their first month of life!

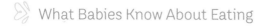

One reason that humans have successfully spread across the world is that they can eat and survive on a wide variety of foods. (Unlike, for example, the koala, which eats mainly eucalyptus leaves.) However, the ability to eat many foods increases the risk of accidentally eating poisonous or harmful foods, or potentially not getting the nutrients needed to be healthy.

Here's how human milk helps with that: because her mother's milk smells and tastes like the foods her mother eats, and it changes all the time, the baby learns that the smells and tastes she's experiencing while nursing are safe and healthy foods.

A baby's early instincts also make her attracted to sweet tastes — a good thing, because human milk tastes very sweet. In fact, drinking a sweetened liquid (such as sugar water) is calming and comforting to a baby experiencing stress — although breastfeeding wins as the most effective calming strategy.

What instincts do babies have when it comes to solid foods? A famous 1928 study by Dr. Clara Davis tried to answer the question about whether babies could choose a healthy diet for themselves. She offered 8- or 9-month-old infants a choice of a large number of different foods, both raw and cooked. The foods were all unprocessed, whole foods served separately — things like cow's milk, vegetables, fruit, meat (including organ meats) and whole grains. She even offered salt, served separately. At each meal, the infants were presented with this array of foods and allowed to pick what they wanted and how much. The infants demonstrated healthy appetites and grew well with their choices.

Two interesting points here: one, the infants showed a lot of fluctuation in the amount of food they ate day by day. One child ate seven eggs in a day (plus other foods) and another consumed four bananas in a day, but on other days, some children ate almost nothing or just small amounts of various foods. (And yes, seven eggs is *a lot* for a baby!) Dr. Davis carefully tracked what the children ate, and despite the big variations from day to day, over a week or so the amount they ate averaged out to plenty of calories and a variety of nutrients to support normal growth.

Second, children with special nutritional needs seemed to know instinctively what they needed to eat. For example, one boy who had been diagnosed with rickets (which is caused by a vitamin D deficiency) was offered cod liver oil (the usual remedy for rickets in 1928) as part of each meal. He was reported to voluntarily drink the cod liver oil every day for about three months. After that time, his vitamin D level was normal and he stopped taking the cod liver oil, even though it was still offered with the other foods.

This research was one of the foundational studies behind the concept of baby-led weaning. One of the goals of baby-led weaning is for babies to learn to pay attention to their own needs in terms of what to eat and how much by listening to what their bodies are saying. Pressuring a baby to eat can disrupt this process, as can restricting the amount of food a baby eats. A 2015 review led by Dr. Netalie Shloim found that the outcomes tended to be the opposite of what parents expected. Babies and toddlers who were pressured to eat more were more likely to be underweight as they got older, and those who had their food restricted were more likely to be overweight.

It's important to note that a key element to the success of baby-led weaning lies in the foods that are offered to the baby. La Leche League's statement on nutrition perhaps captures it best: "a wide variety of foods in as close to their natural state as possible." Therefore, highly processed foods or manufactured foods are problematic not just because they are less likely to promote health, but also because they can confuse a baby's instincts.

Consider, for example, the baby's natural desire for things that taste sweet. If she's being offered "whole foods," this would encourage eating fruit, which provides not just sweetness, but fiber and a range of vitamins and minerals (depending on the fruit). Many ripe vegetables also have a sweet flavor, especially if they are roasted or otherwise cooked. But if the baby is instead offered candy or sugary baked treats, she may well eat it because she's attracted to the sweet flavor. Instead of getting fiber, vitamins

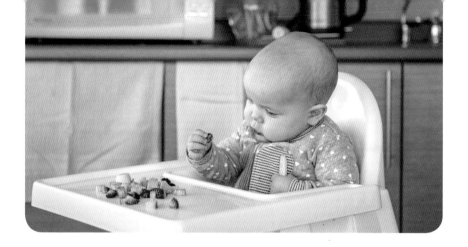

and minerals, though, she only gets the sweetness — an intense sweetness that makes this sugary food even more attractive than naturally sweet foods. So her instincts, which are designed to draw her to the foods she needs to be healthy and to grow, are diverted to foods that won't meet those needs.

If your child is given processed food once in a while, it probably isn't a huge deal. But it's important that most of the time, the foods you offer to your baby are "as close to their natural state as possible."

The Research Is In

Because of the growing popularity of baby-led weaning, a number of studies have been done to see what the outcomes of this approach might be. In 2017, the journal *Current Nutrition Reports* published a study by doctors Amy Brown and Sara Wyn Jones and researcher Hannah Rowan that reviewed the available research. They found that doctors tend to have concerns about the baby-led approach: they worried that babies would choke, that they would not get enough calories or iron, and that parents would feed their babies unsuitable foods, such as french fries.

The review of the research found that these concerns were unwarranted. Babies in the baby-led groups tended to choke at about the same rate as babies in the other groups — around 35 percent would have at least one choking experience. Registered dietitian Jennifer House points out that despite doctors' worries, babies choke more often on non-food items, such as marbles or sand, than on foods. She adds that gagging is common in babies, though, and parents often think their baby is choking. In fact, gagging is an instinctive response in a baby that actually *prevents* choking.

To test doctors' concerns about babies getting enough calories, the same three authors reviewed other studies that had looked at weight gain. They found that babies who started solids with a baby-led approach weighed less, on average, than babies who started solids by being spoon-fed by parents. One study had found that at 24 months, the traditional group weighed (on average) 28 pounds, 6 ounces (12.9 kg), while the baby-led group weighed an average of almost 26 pounds (11.8 kg). This did not indicate a problem, though, because so many babies are overweight. In the traditional, spoon-fed group, 19.2 percent were overweight, but in the baby-led group, only 8 percent were overweight. This can be a significant benefit of baby-led weaning.

One large study Brown, Wyn Jones and Rowan reviewed, known as the Baby-Led Introduction to SolidS (BLISS) study, did not find a significant difference in weight between the traditional group and their modified baby-led group. This could be due to the modifications the researchers recommended, though. The parents in the baby-led group were told to offer foods that were high in iron and protein. It turned out that more than half of them actually spoon-fed their babies infant cereal and other prepared baby foods (possibly because they saw this as a way to give the babies high-iron foods).

Some of the parents using a baby-led approach who were interviewed in another study fed their babies adult foods that were not suitable for babies because they were high in salt, sugar or fat. However, some of the parents using the more traditional approach did the same — the purees they gave their babies initially were healthier, but they added less-healthy foods once their babies got a little older.

Another study Brown, Wyn Jones and Rowan included in their review found that, at 24 months, toddlers were more likely to stop eating when they were full if they had started solids the baby-led way. Those who had been spoon-fed were more prone to keep eating until all the food was gone. This is another positive outcome in favor of baby-led weaning, because that "clean your plate" mentality is more likely to lead to excess weight and obesity.

One of the most important benefits of the baby-led approach may be the attitude toward feeding itself that it can foster. Parents learn to trust their babies to choose the foods and the amounts that they need, and the research found that this trust nurtured a responsive, low-control approach to parenting. In other words, parents respond to a baby's requests for or interests in food, but do not try to pressure the baby to eat more or restrict the amount she can have. Studies have shown that this responsive, low-control approach can reduce the risk of the child later developing an eating disorder, such as anorexia or overeating.

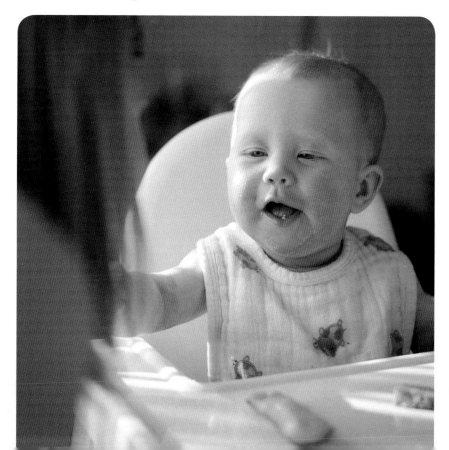

Overall, the review concluded that baby-led weaning is a safe way to introduce solids to a baby's diet with the potential to reduce obesity and future eating disorders.

What if I'm Using Formula?

Much of the research on timing solid foods has been done on breastfed babies. Solid foods shouldn't be started too early, experts say, because these foods will disrupt the gut flora set up by breastfeeding, thus increasing the risk of infection, and their introduction might decrease the mother's milk production. But what if you are feeding formula to your baby, in which case these things would not be an issue? When should formula-fed babies start solid foods?

The formulas on the market today are more complete than those of the 1930s, when Pablum was invented and early solids were recommended, so there is less urgency to add solids to fill in nutritional gaps. Surely that means that in general, formula-feeding parents can reasonably wait until the baby is developmentally ready to self-feed solid foods, right?

Well, it's not entirely clear-cut. A 2012 study by the American Association for Cancer Research found that each month that a baby was exclusively formula-fed increased the baby's risk of pediatric acute lymphoblastic leukemia by 16 percent. (Other studies, which were reviewed in a 2005 meta-analysis by Martin, Gunnell and other researchers, have found that not breastfeeding increases the risk of several childhood cancers, including leukemia, Hodgkin's disease and neuroblastoma.) The researchers from the American Association for Cancer Research suggest that parents who are exclusively feeding formula should start solids as early as possible.

On the other hand, in formula-fed babies, an early start to solid foods increases the risk of later obesity. A 2011 study led by Dr. Susanna Huh found that formula-fed babies were 6.3 times more likely to become obese if they were given solid foods before they were 4 months old compared with

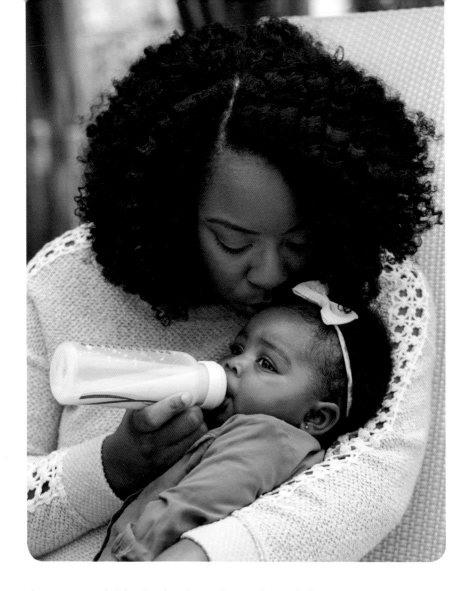

those given solid foods after 4 months. And a study by Diana Cassar-Uhl (which was not yet published at the time of printing) found that babies who were fed any formula were more likely to become obese if given solids before 6 months.

So what's a formula-feeding parent to do? It's tricky. Australian researcher Maureen Minchin has stated that formula-feeding parents may be able to mitigate some of the risks by not sticking to one formula — by giving different ones each day, instead, or even changing them up from feeding to feeding.

Certainly in developmental terms, it makes sense to wait until the baby is showing signs of readiness and allowing him to feed himself. One possible benefit of taking a baby-led approach has not been studied, but here's the thinking: a 2010 study by Li, Fein and Grummer-Strawn compared toddlers who had been fed by bottle (whether the bottle contained formula or human milk) with those who were exclusively breastfed. If given a cup of milk to drink, the bottle-fed toddlers tended to drink the whole thing. The breastfed toddlers would drink as much as they wanted and then stop, even if there was still some left in the cup. A 2011 study led by DiSantis found similar differences in self-regulation.

This is probably because parents giving bottles to babies tend to encourage the baby to drink all of what's in the bottle. If there's half an ounce left, most parents want the baby to drink that last half ounce. Babies being fed at the breast are in control — they stop when they're full.

So if being given bottles increases the risk that a child will develop a pattern of overeating, baby-led weaning could give that child a chance to develop a new pattern: one of responding to her own needs. If the parents can offer solid foods to their baby, with the baby having the freedom to take as much or as little of each food item, this might help to teach that baby to listen to the signals her body is sending her, such as "I'm full now!"

➢→ Back to the Beginning

If you look at the grocery store shelves lined with packages of prepared cereal and jars of baby food, it's natural to assume that these are essential things for feeding your baby — and that they always have been. And certainly if you talk to your parents or grandparents, you'll hear stories about introducing solids to babies who were just a few weeks old. But if you look at the bigger picture, you'll see that the past 80 years have been a departure from the long history of how babies were fed. Until the 1900s, babies were fed family foods around the middle of their first year, and they mostly picked up the food and fed themselves — or licked it off mom's or dad's fingers. What might seem like a radical new idea or scary trend to some is really a return to the feeding patterns that existed throughout human history.

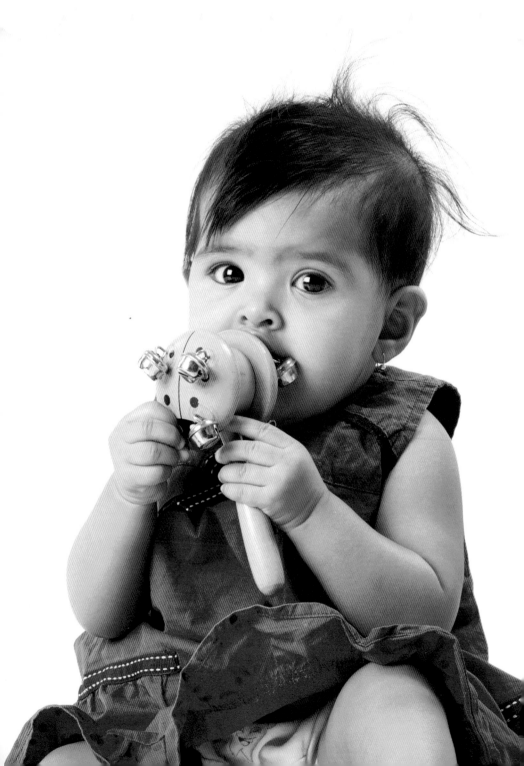

3

Getting Ready

From birth, your baby has been learning about food and eating, and the skills she's developed and experiences she's had with feeding will prepare her for starting solids. In this chapter, you'll learn about the normal process of infant development in terms of feeding and how a baby-led approach to solids fits in.

Baby-Led Feeding from the Start

People used to think that newborns had to be taught how to eat. But nature has a better plan: babies are born with great instincts about feeding, and the parents' role is to support those instincts instead of fight them.

Beginning at the Breast

For a newborn baby, being able to get food is critical. He has spent the past nine months happily taking in the needed nutrients through his umbilical cord, but now that he's born, for the first time he will need to work for his supper. The good news is that he has all the inborn skills and knowledge he needs to make that happen.

For a long time, medical professionals and parenting instructors have been saying that breastfeeding is a learned skill, something new parents (often with the help of nurses or lactation consultants) need to teach their baby. It turns out they're wrong about that. Babies, like other mammals, are born knowing how to find and latch onto the breast. Then why do so many mothers and babies have problems getting breastfeeding going? Well, there are two reasons.

One reason is that the baby may be affected by medications given to the mother during labor and birth. These drugs can make the baby groggy and disoriented. A video from 1987 by Swedish researcher Anne-Marie Widstrom shows how newborn babies placed on their mothers' bellies could crawl to their mothers' breasts, find the nipple, latch on and feed effectively within an hour of being born. The video also shows that babies who had been exposed to medications during labor, including epidural anesthetics, weren't nearly as successful at doing this as the babies who hadn't. They were unable to find their mothers' breasts or nipples, they would attempt to latch and then drop the nipple without sucking or they would simply lie on their mothers' bodies without moving toward the breasts.

As described in the book *Impact of Birthing Practices on Breastfeeding* by Linda Smith and Mary Kroeger, several factors influence how labor drugs can affect a baby's abilities: the length of time that the baby was exposed to the medication (an epidural given over many hours would have a bigger effect than an epidural given right before the baby was delivered by cesarean section, for example), the dosage

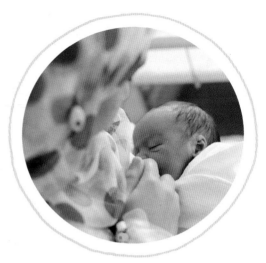

and the type of medication (some have more of an effect on a baby's ability to latch and feed than others). While the drugs may inhibit the baby's abilities at first, usually the effects wear off within a few days and the baby will be much more effective at latching and feeding.

The trick is to keep the mother's milk production going and to find ways to feed the baby that don't interfere with the breastfeeding skills he'll need. To ensure milk production, the milk in the breasts needs to be removed frequently and effectively. In the first few days, while the mother is producing colostrum (a concentrated form of milk that helps to "clean out" the baby's system and provides the baby with antibodies and essential nutrients), hand-expressing the milk usually works if the baby is not latching. After the volume of milk increases, a pump can be more effective. The baby can be fed with a spoon (which is especially helpful when feeding colostrum, because the quantities are small), a syringe (with the needle removed, of course), a tube attached to a parent's finger or a small open cup. If the baby will latch but doesn't feed well, a tube can be used at the breast.

The second reason behind breastfeeding problems is that mothers often

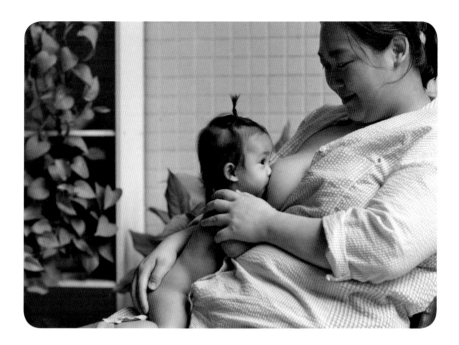

put the baby in a position that is abnormal for him, so he can't do what his instincts would tell him to do. Those instincts work best when the baby is in a position that has been described by several experts as follows: the mother gets into a comfortable, semi-reclined position, with the baby lying tummy-down on the mother's chest or abdomen. The mother can support the baby and help as needed. The baby uses his feet to crawl and push himself into position to latch onto the breast, usually coming down on the nipple from above.

Mothers are often advised to sit up straight to breastfeed. This can work if the baby is positioned vertically, with her head against the mother's upper chest and her bottom supported against the mother's belly. If the baby is hungry, she soon begins to bob her head around, throwing her head back to orient herself by looking at her mother's face and then moving down toward one breast or the other (sometimes quite vigorously). The mother's task is to support the baby and follow her movements as she moves to the breast and latches on.

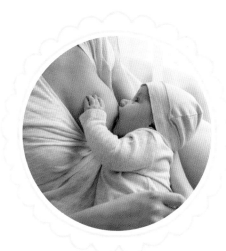

Usually, though, mothers are not only told to sit up, but also to hold the baby horizontally and help him latch on (likely because the person providing these instructions believes the baby has to learn how to breast-feed). This often means pushing the baby toward the breast and trying to get the nipple in his mouth as he opens wide. For the baby, this can be very confusing. He has a whole set of built-in behaviors to seek out and latch onto the breast, but in this horizontal position, he can't do any of them. He expects to latch onto the nipple from above, but now that he's positioned below or beside the breast, he can't do that either. Many breastfeeding problems can be prevented or solved by allowing the baby to follow his instincts, find the breast and self-attach.

When a newborn baby starts to feed, he won't get much milk. For the first couple of days, breastfeeding mothers produce colostrum in small amounts. Within a few days, the volume of milk begins to increase, and the baby's sucking skills develop to deal with these changes.

As breastfeeding becomes established, the baby will follow a typical pattern. At first he uses fast, short sucks that help him get the small amount of milk that is available while stimulating the let-down reflex in the mother that causes the milk to flow. Once the milk has let down, the baby will start using longer, slower sucks with pauses when his mouth is wide open. This change in sucking shows that the baby is getting substantial amounts of milk, and it requires different muscles and different coordination with breathing.

Periodically during the feeding, the baby will pause. Newborns pause more often than older babies, and they may use these pauses to rest, catch up with breathing or control the amount of food they take in. Sometimes parents worry about these pauses and try to nudge the baby to keep on feeding, but the pauses are important. Patience is a valuable skill when you are feeding a baby.

You'll probably notice similarities between baby-led breastfeeding and baby-led weaning: baby-led breastfeeding lets a baby use her instincts to find and latch onto her mother's breast and listen to her inner cues about how often and how long to feed; baby-led weaning allows a baby to demonstrate her readiness for solid foods and listen to her inner cues about which of the offered foods to eat and how much to eat.

Beginning at the Bottle

How might this idea of letting a baby lead the feeding apply to a bottle-fed baby? No, babies aren't born with instincts related to bottles, but parents can be aware of their baby's feeding skills and be responsive to his needs.

Many infant feeding experts recommend "paced bottle feeding." The first step is to change how the bottle-fed baby is held. Just as mothers often try to breastfeed in a position that is less than helpful, parents often put babies in an unhelpful position for bottle feeding, with the baby lying on his back in the crook of a parent's arm and the bottle held vertically.

Paced bottle feeding requires a different position. The parent supports the baby with one arm, so that he's in a semi-sitting position, and then holds the bottle horizontally. Why do this? Well, if the bottle is vertical and the baby is lying on his back, milk will automatically drip out of the nipple into the baby's mouth thanks to gravity. But if the bottle is horizontal, the baby will have to suck to get milk out of the nipple — just like a breastfed baby does. This position helps the baby learn better sucking skills and, just as importantly, lets him control the amount of milk he takes in. When he stops sucking, milk will stop flowing (or will at least slow down).

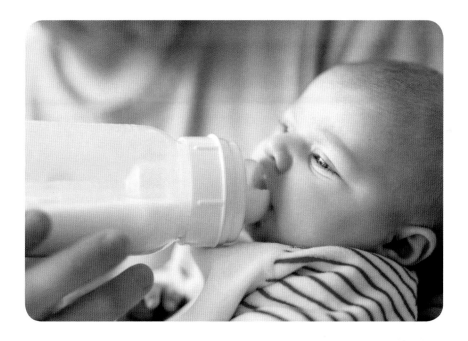

This doesn't always work perfectly with very young babies. For these babies, the feeling of the firm bottle nipple stimulates the sucking reflex, so as long as the nipple is in the baby's mouth, she'll keep sucking and getting milk. That's where the paced part of the approach comes in. The parent giving the bottle carefully watches the baby for signs that she wants to stop. That could be trying to turn her head away from the nipple, trying to lean away from the nipple, using her hands to push the bottle away or other actions that indicate she wants to stop. At that point, the parent can remove the bottle from the baby's mouth or tip the bottom of the bottle down so that the milk is no longer flowing into the nipple part.

The baby might be done or might just want to take a little break. Just as a breastfed baby pauses while feeding, bottle-fed babies need pauses, too. The parent should wait a little bit and let the baby rest, or maybe try burping the baby in case she has swallowed some air. If the baby seems to be looking for the bottle again after a minute or two, or begins to fuss, the parent can touch the nipple to the baby's lips again and see if she takes it. The bottle nipple shouldn't be pushed into the baby's mouth. Let her grasp it.

If she isn't interested, even if there is an ounce or half an ounce left in the bottle, the feeding should be over. The temptation to try to get all the milk into the baby might be strong, but it's better for the baby to control how much she takes.

ᐁᐧ Feeding Skills

The skills needed to self-feed are more complicated than they might seem at first glance. To feed effectively, your baby has had to master several different things, whether he was breastfeeding or bottle feeding. To eat solid foods, your baby will need some new abilities.

ᐁᐧ Tongue Coordination

While sucking at the breast or the bottle, a baby uses his tongue. The actual movements and effects are different between these two feeding methods, but the tongue's role is vital. The next stage in feeding skills involves being able to use the tongue to move food from the front of the mouth to the back.

We adults do this all the time without thinking about it: you pick up a tasty-looking morsel on your fork and put it in your mouth, near the front and on top of your tongue. If the food is soft and dissolves easily, you may hold it there briefly and then move it toward your throat. If the food needs chewing, you'll move it toward your teeth and then, once it's mashed enough, toward your throat. You unconsciously coordinate all of this with your breathing, but when you think about it, it's a fairly complicated series of movements.

The breastfed baby uses her tongue in a particular way. When she latches onto the breast, her tongue covers her bottom jaw and lower lip and cups the breast. As she begins to suck, the back part of her tongue (nearest her throat) moves up, compressing the breast and nipple, and then down, creating a vacuum that helps to pull out the milk.

The bottle-fed baby uses his tongue a bit differently. The bottle nipple sits at the front of his mouth; it doesn't fill his mouth the way the breast and nipple do. He doesn't bring his tongue as far forward and doesn't compress the nipple, but he can press his tongue against the end of the nipple to slow down the flow if it becomes too much. This difference in movement is why some babies who have been drinking from a bottle have a hard time going back to the breast.

The tongue movements used for breastfeeding and bottle feeding are different from those needed for eating solid foods. That's why when young babies are spoon-fed cereal or other solids, they tend to push the food right back out. Some of the food may end up staying in their mouths, but that's more of an accident than anything else. Their tongues are not yet ready to manage solid foods. But by the middle of the first year, babies become more capable of using their tongues in other ways. They can take food and move it to the back of their mouths or to the jaws or teeth for mashing or chewing.

Tongue-Tied Babies • We all have a membrane, called a frenulum, under our tongues, which attaches the tongue to the bottom of our mouths. In some babies, the frenulum is short and tight, restricting the movement of the tongue enough that the baby can't breastfeed or bottle feed effectively. This is called tongue-tie, or ankyloglossia. In some cases, the 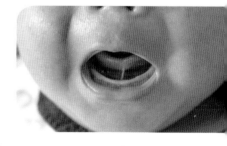 baby may be able to breastfeed, but the mother's nipples become very sore because of the abnormal action of the baby's tongue. Often, tongue-tie is treated by cutting the frenulum with scissors or burning it with a laser. This diagnosis is not always easy to make, and the treatments are controversial, but there is no question that this is an issue for some babies. It can also affect the baby when it comes to eating solid foods.

If the movement of the baby's tongue is restricted, she may not be able to smoothly move the food to her gums for chewing or to her throat. The effort it takes to do this might make it hard to coordinate breathing at the same time. She might try swallowing the food before it's been sufficiently chewed or push the food back out because she can't get it to her throat. It's something to watch for if your baby was previously diagnosed with tongue-tie but the frenulum was not released, or if you think the frenulum might have grown back.

Digestion and Taste

At the same time a baby's tongue becomes capable of moving food around, digestive enzymes begin to appear in his saliva to help break down the food as it is chewed or moved around in the mouth. These enzymes are not really necessary when the baby's diet is primarily breast milk, which already contains enzymes to help with digestion. With solid foods, though, digestion begins in the mouth.

If a baby is breastfeeding, he is also developing a sense of taste that will direct his food preferences. Breastfeeding prepares a baby for solid foods by introducing a variety of tastes. Human milk picks up flavors from all the foods in the breastfeeding mother's diet. Some flavors are so strong that you can smell them in pumped milk — try eating a lot of garlic one day and hand-expressing some milk the next day; you'll be able to smell the garlic. (And research has shown that most babies respond very positively to garlicky milk and tend to consume more of it.) But even more subtle flavors come through in a mother's milk, and they teach the baby about how safe foods taste and what his family eats. Researchers have found that when breastfeeding mothers eat plenty of vegetables, for example, the baby will be more interested in eating vegetables and will eat larger quantities of them when solid foods are started.

 ## Motor Skills

Another skill that develops around the same time as tongue coordination is the ability to pick things up fairly reliably and transfer them to the mouth. The baby begins by picking things up with her whole hand, fingers wrapped around whatever it is. At first, she is pretty uncoordinated. You've probably seen a baby — if not your own baby — try to pick up a piece of food and hit her cheeks or chin with it rather than get it in her wide-open mouth. Or she grabs a piece of food but puts her fist in her mouth instead

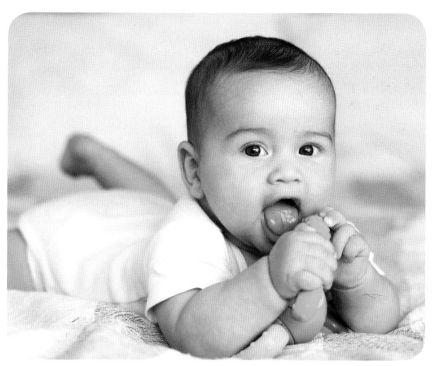

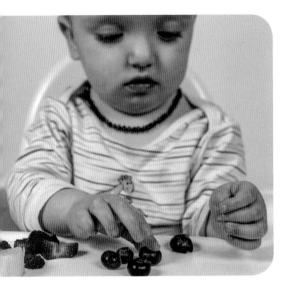

of the part of the food projecting from her fist. Or she opens her hand too soon, and the food falls out of her hand on the way to her mouth. It's a messy process. With time, these skills improve, and soon the baby becomes quite efficient at getting food to her mouth.

The next skill is called the pincer grip. This usually appears somewhere between 8 and 12 months as a baby learns to use her thumb and forefinger to pick up small pieces of food — a pea, a little cube of cheese or even a crumb from a cracker. She couldn't possibly have done this a month ago, but now she can transfer that single pea from her high-chair tray to her mouth. This skill will be useful for many aspects of eating.

From here, the baby will figure out how to use utensils — first a spoon, later a fork and much later still a knife — to pick up and move foods to her mouth. We do these things all the time, but the movements are more complex than we think. The baby has to manage dipping the spoon into the food, moving it to her mouth while keeping it (more or less) horizontal so that the food doesn't fall off, correctly judging the distance to get it to her mouth (which is not the same as putting her fingers in her mouth) and, finally, once the food is in her mouth, tipping the spoon so the food falls off. Sure, we adults can do this practically in our sleep, but for a baby there's a lot to learn.

All babies will eventually develop these skills, no matter how they are fed solids. The baby who is spoon-fed by a parent at 6 months will at some point start insisting on picking up food from her high-chair tray. The baby who has developed a pincer grip will use it to pick up pieces of lint from the carpet if there are no peas available to practice on. But baby-led weaning works *with* the baby's developing skills rather than around them.

⊳→ Signs of Readiness

Remember Isla and Lisa? When Lisa was wondering whether Isla was ready to start solids, she turned to her La Leche League Leader, who provided her with these guidelines for readiness:

1. The baby is able to sit up comfortably without support. This makes it possible for her to pick up food and put it in her mouth and be in control of the process.

2. The baby has the dexterity needed to pick up objects and move them to her mouth.

3. The baby no longer has the tongue extrusion reflex seen in younger babies. To eat solids, she needs to be able to move the food from the front of her mouth to the back, where it is swallowed.

4. The baby shows interest in food, perhaps reaching for food from a parent's plate or watching intently as a parent eats.

All four of these signs need to be present before solid foods are started.

Of course, even a baby with all these signs present might not actually be ready to eat. This is an important part of baby-led weaning: you follow the baby's lead.

Jenna's 7-month-old baby girl, Ahsoka, seemed to have all the signs of readiness for solid foods. She sat up well on her own, liked to reach out for items and was doing a good job of picking up fairly small things.

"I decided to give it a try," Jenna says. She took some guacamole she had prepared for the family and set it on a plate on the table, holding Ahsoka on her lap, where she could reach it. Sure enough, Ahsoka reached out and scooped up the little lump of avocado mixture and popped it in her mouth. It quickly went downhill. Ahsoka started to swallow the guacamole but then gagged, fussed and eventually vomited not just the guacamole, but also all the milk she had drunk over the last hour or so.

"I was drenched," says Jenna. "I literally had to change my clothes and hers." She decided to wait a bit longer to offer Ahsoka solid foods.

If you give your baby the opportunity to try some food and he puts it in his mouth but then promptly spits it out, or he gives some tentative chews while holding it and then drops it on the floor, maybe he is trying to tell you:

- I'm not really ready for solid foods.
- I don't like that particular food.
- My coordination isn't that great yet, and I accidentally dropped the food or pushed it out of my mouth. Can I try again?

There's only one way to know: try again. The baby who accidentally dropped the food will probably respond eagerly to your offer of another piece. The baby who isn't ready to start eating might play with it for a while. The baby who doesn't like the taste might push it away; try a different food and see if you get a better response.

Here's another baby: 5-month-old Matthew has always been advanced in his physical development. He rolled over at 6 weeks, both from front to back and back to front. He started crawling at 4 months and could soon get around pretty quickly. Lately he has been showing a lot of interest in what his parents are eating. One day, while he was sitting on his dad's lap, he reached up and tried to grab the forkful of food that his father, David, was about to eat. "I pretty much had to wrestle it away from him," David says.

Matthew's mother, Suzanne, knew about the recommendations that solid foods should be delayed until 6 months, but she couldn't help wondering if Matthew might be ready. Should she wait?

Then one evening, Matthew was playing with toys across the room when Suzanne filled the dog's dish with food. As she went to put the container of dog food away, Matthew scooted across the room and started eating out of the dog's bowl (much to the consternation of the dog). Suzanne was horrified. She called her doctor's office, worried that her son had been poisoned. The doctor called her back and actually thought it was pretty funny.

"No," she told Suzanne. "A little dog food won't hurt him. But I think he's trying to tell you something: he's ready to start solid foods."

The next day, Suzanne set Matthew up in his high chair with some pieces of banana. He happily gobbled them up and looked around for more. Yes: he was ready.

Knowing the signs of readiness will help you in planning a start, but in the end it's up to your baby — and every baby is a little different. Matthew's sister, for example, had no interest in solid foods until she was 9 months old.

The Non-Indicators

There are some false signs of readiness that can confuse some parents.

Weight Gain • Many parents hear that if a baby has doubled his birth weight, or if he weighs more than 14 pounds (6.4 kg), it's time to start solid foods.

Many babies double their birth weight at some point between 4 and 6 months, so this "guideline" may bring the baby into the recommended timetable for starting solids. But a smaller baby (such as a premature baby) might double his birth weight at a much earlier age, even though his system is likely to be ready for solids later than average.

The 14-pound guideline is similar. If a baby is born weighing 7 pounds (3.2 kg), which was the average weight for a newborn a generation ago, that baby will typically have doubled his weight to — surprise! — 14 pounds by between 4 and 6 months. (Today's average newborn weight is 7 pounds, 13 ounces (3.5 kg) in Canada and 7 pounds, 8 ounces (3.4 kg) in the U.S., so the weight guideline would need to shift anyway.) And of course, this guideline only applies to an average baby. A baby born weighing 11 pounds

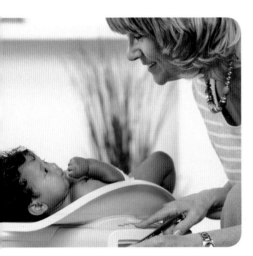

(5.0 kg) is likely to hit 14 pounds by 8 weeks, which is much too early for solid foods.

It's not so much that achieving this particular weight gain indicates readiness for solid foods. It's simply that it tends to happen (on average) around the middle of the first year, when babies are usually ready.

Slowed Weight Gain • At every well-baby check, the doctor plots the baby's weight on a chart to see if she is following the expected growth pattern. For breastfed babies, weight gain during the first two or three months tends to be a bit faster than it is for formula-fed babies. But at around 4 months, the rate of weight gain usually slows down. The breastfed babies are still gaining weight, but not as quickly as they were in those early months. The rate slows even more during the second half of the first year.

Formula-fed babies tend to gain weight at a more consistent rate throughout the year. There is some slowing, but not as much as for breastfed babies. Unfortunately, that more consistent pattern of weight gain is linked to childhood and adult obesity.

You've probably seen a growth chart: these charts have gently curved lines, and the baby's weight is expected to (roughly) follow the curve he starts out on. If a baby's recorded weight starts to fall below the curve, then a doctor may become concerned that the baby is not getting enough to eat.

Until recently, the growth charts used by most North American doctors were based primarily on formula-fed babies. This wasn't because of any prejudice against breastfed babies; rather, it was because most babies were formula-fed when the charts were made. These charts, however, created some problems for parents of breastfed babies. When the pattern of weight gain for breastfed babies was compared with the curves that were based on formula-fed babies, the breastfed babies seemed to be faltering. Doctors would look at the charts and decide that the breastfed babies weren't getting enough to eat; if they didn't suggest formula supplementation (or if the parents resisted that idea), they'd often suggest starting solid foods.

The World Health Organization (WHO) came to the rescue by doing a large study with groups of babies from several countries around the world. Their study included only breastfed babies who started solid foods at the recommended 6 months. The new curves on the graph flattened out by around 4 months and had a lower average weight at 1 year. This growth pattern is linked to better overall health and lower rates of excess weight and obesity later in life.

So if your baby is breastfeeding and your doctor suggests that she might need solid foods to "get her back on the curve," you can ask whether the WHO growth charts are being used. If not, ask your doctor to use them instead to get a better assessment.

> The WHO growth charts are available online at who.int/childgrowth/standards/weight_for_age/en/.

Teething • Sometimes people tell parents that if their babies are getting teeth, it's time to start "real food." The behaviors common with teething — chewing on fingers and toys or fussing during feedings — can also be interpreted as the baby being ready for solid foods. The problem with using

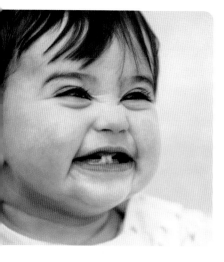

the arrival of teeth as a guideline is that some babies are born with teeth already in their mouths, and other babies don't get them until they are more than 1 year old. This makes them a pretty unreliable gauge for starting solids.

If your baby doesn't have teeth at 6 or 7 months, will he be able to manage eating the foods he can pick up himself? How can he chew or bite without teeth? Parents sometimes worry about this when deciding whether to use the baby-led approach.

Fortunately, babies are very capable of gumming reasonably soft foods enough to swallow them. (If you have ever been bitten by a toothless baby, you know how strong their jaws are!)

How Long Is Too Long?

If your baby is not interested in eating at 6 months, it's not a big deal. But let's say he's still uninterested at 7 months, then 8 months. At what point does it become a concern?

Registered dietitian Jennifer House says that she finds most babies are interested in eating by 8 months, even if they are not at 6. She encourages parents to start offering food at 6 months, but not to be concerned if it takes four to six weeks before the baby actually starts eating. "There's a saying you sometimes hear that 'food before one is just for fun,' and while that is sort of true, babies do need the extra nutrition by around six months. Getting iron is especially important for breastfed babies, but they also need zinc and extra fats," House says.

If a breastfed baby is 8 months old and is still uninterested in solids, House recommends having the baby's iron level tested. If needed, the baby can be given supplements. "Babies who are low in iron or zinc may also have lowered appetites," she adds. That means that even though they need the extra nutrients, they don't have the desire to eat solids in order to get them. Instead, they are content just to nurse. House suggests that once these babies are supplemented and get up to normal levels of iron and zinc, they often begin showing interest in solid foods.

Most formulas have iron added, so making sure the baby is getting enough iron is less of a concern for formula-feeding parents. However, for formula-fed babies, adding some solids by about 6 months is generally recommended. There are many micronutrients — nutrients that are needed in small amounts — that may become depleted in babies who are only fed formula for a long time. Also, as mentioned in the previous chapter, at least one study shows that the risk of developing certain childhood cancers increases when solids are delayed for formula-fed babies. Lastly, it's important for those babies to begin experiencing different tastes and textures in food. Eating these foods at a developmentally appropriate time helps prepare the baby to enjoy a variety of foods throughout his life.

⊳→ Setting the Table

Today's the day. Your baby is showing all the signs of readiness and you've decided it's time to offer solid foods.

Bring out your fine china and best silverware . . . just kidding!

For your baby's first attempts at eating solids, there's no need for anything special. He can just sit on your lap at the table and eat something from your plate or out

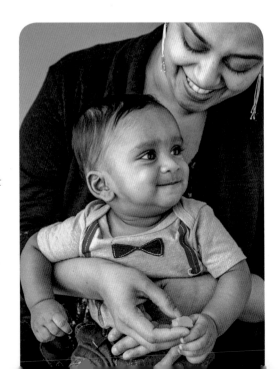

of your hand. In fact, being on your lap can be helpful — he'll be reassured by your closeness as he embarks on his new eating adventure. But as your baby transitions to regular solid meals, you'll want to arrange some kind of dining setup for him.

High Chairs

There are two types of high chairs (with many variations). Some are designed so that the chair sits beside (or slightly under) a standard dining table. Your baby's food needs to be set on a plate at the table. The other kind of high chair has its own tray. You can put the food on a plate or bowl on the tray, or put food on the tray itself.

Both have their own advantages and disadvantages. The baby in the first type of chair can sit at the dining table with the rest of the family, but he is more likely to make a mess. The tray-type high chair contains the mess a bit better, but the baby can only sit near the dining table, not right at it.

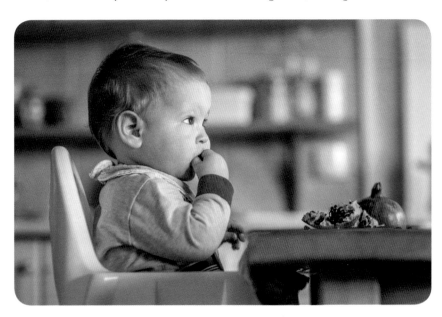

Plates

Non-breakable is the golden rule for your baby's first plates, since there's a good chance they'll be thrown on the floor more than once in the next few months. One useful feature to look for is some kind of suction cup on the bottom. These suction cups don't make the plates impossible for your baby to lift up and throw (as your baby will demonstrate soon enough), but

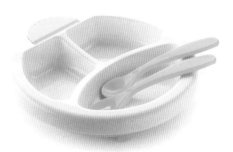

they may slow things down enough for you to grab the plate before it goes.

A popular design for parents using a baby-led approach is the divided plate. Having different foods in each section seems to appeal to babies and lets them feel more in control. It can also help you in planning the meal, as you think about what to put in each section.

The first time you offer your baby solids may feel like a big deal, or it may feel like just a small step in your baby's development. Either way, the next few chapters are designed to help you make the best decisions on what foods to offer your baby.

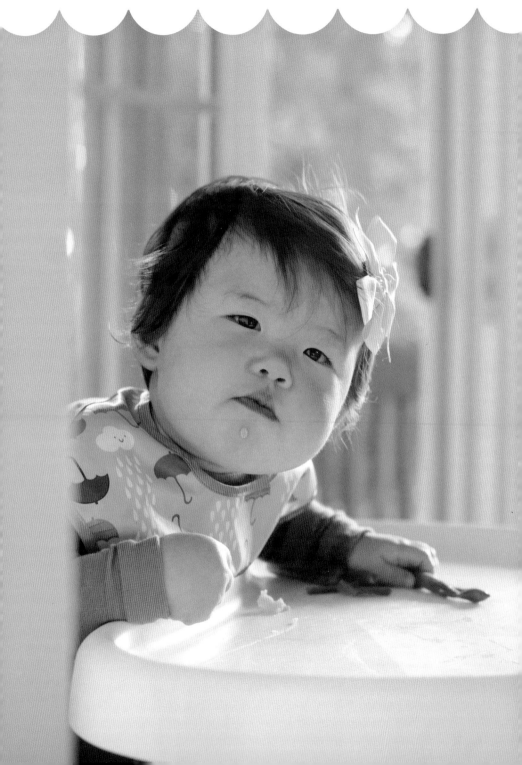

4

Starting Baby-Led Weaning

Providing "real" foods rather than purees means you have many more options — and sometimes that can be daunting. In this chapter you will get some ideas about nutritious foods that are likely to appeal to babies, learn how to prepare them and learn how to deal with some of the common concerns parents have when their babies start eating solids (such as the baby gagging and choking).

⤳ Baby-Led Weaning for Breastfed Babies

You may have heard the saying, "Food before one is just for fun." That's not strictly true: by 6 months, most breastfed babies will need the additional iron and protein that solid foods can supply. But breast milk should still provide most of your baby's nutrition: solid foods should add to your baby's diet, but not replace the milk.

For that reason, it's recommended that your baby breastfeeds before he eats his solids, at least for the first three or four months after he starts solid foods. This will help ensure that your eager eater doesn't fill up on so many solid foods that he won't nurse as much, which could increase the risk of reducing the breastfeeding mother's milk production.

Early on, there's no need to plan meals with solid foods at set times, although it's ideal if your baby can share his meal with the rest of the family. If you have a large and active family and your baby is just starting solids, it may be easier to pick a quiet time and let the baby explore his food on his own. As for when to offer solids after breastfeeding, you should choose a time when your baby has just nursed but is still awake and interested in exploring. For some babies, that time will be predictable and for others it will not be, so watch for a good moment.

Even as a baby begins adding new foods to his diet, the breastfeeding mother should expect to continue breastfeeding in response to the baby's cues. As the baby gets older, nursing becomes as much about comforting, calming and reassuring as it is about food and nutrition, so don't be surprised if your baby wants to nurse quite frequently at times. And don't hesitate to offer the breast even if your baby isn't asking: your baby will let you know if he's not interested at the moment.

⤳ Baby-Led Weaning for Bottle-Fed Babies

It's not as crucial to bottle-feed before you give your baby solid foods because if the baby rejects the bottle after eating solids, there's no effect on the mother's milk production. That's true even if you are giving pumped breast milk in a bottle — the pumping controls the amount of milk the mother makes, not the amount the baby takes.

However, at the beginning it's still a good idea to give the breast milk or formula before solid foods most of the time. Milk or formula should continue to provide most of the baby's nutrition for the second half of the first year.

When feeding with a bottle, practice the paced bottle feeding technique described in chapter 3 (pages 58–60) and follow the baby's cues about when he wants to drink and for how long.

⤙→ The First Meal

There are a couple of things to consider as you decide what to give your baby as her first food.

If there is a tendency toward allergies in the baby's family, you might want to read the chapter on allergies (chapter 6) next. But for now, just remember that the key is to offer one food at a time, so that you know if your baby turns out to be allergic to something. If you are serving your family mixed vegetables, pick out just one type to offer to your baby. Skip the pancakes because they contain too many possible allergens, and instead choose a single food, such as banana or baked sweet potato.

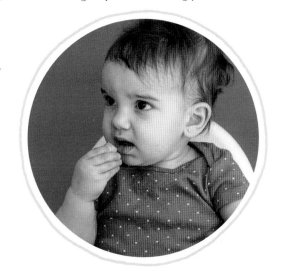

Similarly, if your family is following a specific diet — say you're vegan, vegetarian or paleo — you might want to review chapter 5, which talks about special diets.

If your family doesn't have allergies or dietary restrictions, you might not be too worried about these factors. Just take a look at what your family is eating for your next meal, and see if there is something suitable. Do you have some steamed mixed vegetables on the menu? Let some cool to room temperature, and put those on your baby's plate or high-chair tray. Beef stew? Try offering her a piece of stewed meat with a well-braised piece of carrot. Oatmeal with blueberries? Make it without any added sugars (including honey or syrup), and scoop out a portion for the baby before you add your sweeteners. Let it cool to room temperature, when it will usually thicken, to make it easier for your baby to pick up.

Human milk is quite sweet, so many breastfed babies like to start with fruit, such as banana, apple or peach. However, breastfed babies have typically been exposed to quite a few flavors based on what their mothers eat, so things like sweet potato, avocado and other vegetables are also popular if they are foods the breastfeeding mother eats frequently. Formula has a blander taste, so formula-fed babies often do well starting with foods like cubes of baked or steamed potatoes or oatmeal.

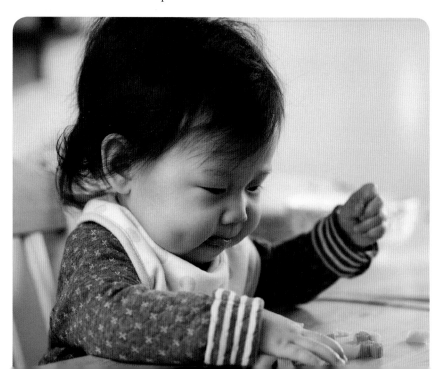

Popular First Foods

- Sticks or cubes of banana
- Cubes of ripe peach
- Cubes of ripe mango
- Cubes of ripe avocado
- Sticks of baked sweet potato
- Thick oatmeal, unsweetened and cooled to room temperature

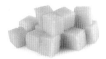

First Food No-Nos

- Anything fried
- Anything with added salt or sugar
- Anything spicy
- Foods that a baby might choke on (grapes, raw carrots, hot dogs, nuts, etc.)
- Processed meats (sandwich meats, pepperoni, hot dogs, etc.)
- Honey (it may contain botulism spores, which can make babies under 1 year old very ill)

This doesn't mean that you need to stick with these foods — obviously one of your goals in feeding solids is to introduce your baby to a variety of tastes and foods. But for your baby's first try at solids, it often helps to give her something that tastes at least a bit familiar.

So you've offered your baby a solid food. What happens next? Well, that depends on the baby.

She'll probably want to explore a bit. She might gobble it up. She might play with it. She might do a little bit of both. She might eat it and want more. Or she might bring it to her lips and reject it completely. Whatever happens, enjoy the process.

Usually, parents do just one meal a day of solids for a week or two. Then they move to two meals a day for a few weeks and then to three meals a day if it's going well. But there is no rush. If your baby is not interested, you might wait a few days before offering solids again. Proceed at the pace that seems to work best for you and your baby. One caveat: if you are breastfeeding, remember that you want to maintain your milk production, so make sure to breastfeed before feeding your baby solid foods at least until your baby is 9 or 10 months old.

At this early stage, portions are likely to be small. Your baby might only eat a teaspoon of food at each meal. That's fine. Remember that one important goal of baby-led solids is to let the baby decide how much he wants to eat. He's learning to respond to his body's signals, and this is setting him up for a lifetime of healthy eating. Some babies, of course, will eat more — and some a lot more. These are all normal variations.

Keep Offering

You may find that there are some foods your baby usually rejects. In the 1928 study described in chapter 2, Dr. Clara Davis found the same thing: she reported that sometimes a child would put a piece of food into his mouth, promptly spit it out and not pick it up again. Each child had his or her own favorite foods as well as foods that were never or almost never eaten.

But over the course of the study — which was six months — Dr. Davis found that children often started eating foods that they had previously ignored or rejected. Other studies have found the same thing: children's tastes seem to change over time.

The recommendation? Keep offering. You don't need to offer a lot, and it's not helpful to try to force your baby to eat a food she has ignored or rejected, but just keep putting it on the plate from time to time. One 2007 study of 7-month-old babies found that offering a rejected food at least eight times seemed to make that food as acceptable as foods the babies liked the first time. And the effects lasted – nine months later, that once-rejected food was still readily eaten. As well, seeing parents or other family members eating particular foods can help encourage a baby to give the foods a try.

⤳ Gagging and Choking

Choking is probably the number one worry parents have about baby-led weaning. (And according to research, it's the number one worry for doctors, too.) The good news is that research has shown that babies using the baby-led approach are no more likely to choke than those following the spoon-feeding method of introducing solids. The concerns come from a time when babies were being given foods at a much younger age. A baby who is only 6 weeks old needs his solid food pureed because he doesn't have same the tongue control or ability to chew that he will at 6 months.

Babies have an amazing gag reflex. It's much more sensitive than an adult's. So if your baby manages to gnaw off a fairly big chunk of sweet potato or some other food, that gag reflex will kick in. You'll hear her cough and sputter as she clears the food out of her throat, but then she'll be fine. Remember, if your baby is coughing, she's not choking — she's just doing what she needs to do to clear the food from her throat.

Another way to differentiate between gagging and choking is as follows: babies who are gagging often have red faces and make a lot of noise (mostly coughing); babies who are choking may start to turn blue, especially around the lips, and will be silent and unable to make noise.

Certain foods are more dangerous and can cause choking: foods that are firm and round (such as whole grapes) can more easily block a baby's throat and are tough for the baby to dislodge through coughing; hard foods in chunks that are small enough can get into a baby's throat and stick there (such as raw apple or carrots); and some soft foods, such as peanut butter or cheese, can stick together strongly enough that they may also be a risk.

Common Choking Hazards

- Hot dogs
- Whole grapes
- Raw baby carrots
- Raw apple slices
- Hard candy
- Popcorn
- Nuts

What can you do? First, never leave a baby alone while he's eating. It's good for meals to be sociable anyway — your baby benefits from having you around to talk to and provide an example of happy, healthy eating. And in case something does go wrong, you'll be right there.

Second, take a course in infant CPR. This is recommended for all parents anyway, as it prepares them to deal with a variety of situations in which a baby may be choking or in need of resuscitation. (The truth is that babies choke more often on other objects — such as stones, marbles or parts of toys — than on food.)

Third, avoid the foods listed on the previous page. Some can be easily modified: whole grapes can be cut into quarters, and carrots and apples can be shredded, cut into small pieces or cooked until soft. Offer peanut butter or soft cheese in small blobs or spread them on a piece of pita or a soft cracker. If you want to give your baby some popcorn, break it into small pieces and don't give him the hard part of the kernel. Candy and hot dogs are best avoided altogether.

With most other foods, you don't need to worry — your baby will manage them just fine.

➢→ Building Meals

Once your baby is eating more than one food at a time, you'll be getting into planning meals, although, as you'll see, the phrase "planning meals" is a bit of an exaggeration. You don't need to be Martha Stewart to feed your baby, and there's no need to make your baby's mealtimes complicated. Nevertheless, there are basic components that every meal you offer your baby should have:

- A source of iron
- A source of protein
- A source of healthy fat
- At least one vegetable
- At least one fruit

Keeping these categories in mind will help ensure you're offering options that meet your baby's nutritional needs. But again, this doesn't need to be complicated. As long as you're eating healthy, balanced meals, your baby can have some of what you're having. In most cases, your family's meals can be adapted to make them appropriate for your baby, and easy finger foods can be offered to supplement meals when needed.

For example, let's say your family is having fried chicken, mashed potatoes and salad for dinner plus ice cream for dessert. How can you turn this into a meal for your baby?

Let's start with the chicken. If you peel off the fried coating, the meat underneath should be fine to offer. You can cut some into small pieces for your baby. Now you've got a source of protein with some iron.

Now for the potatoes. There are a couple of options here. You could put aside some of the boiled potatoes before mashing them, cut them into small, soft chunks and let them cool to room temperature. Easy! Or, you could mash the potatoes with just a little milk and butter so that they are still pretty chunky and set those aside for your baby. Then mash and season the rest of the potatoes as you normally would for the older eaters.

If you're in the mood to get fancier (and pack in more nutrition), boil or steam some cauliflower as you prepare the potatoes, mash the cauliflower with some of the potatoes and set the mixture aside. Then take half a can of drained, rinsed white beans and put them in a blender with enough milk so that the resulting puree can act as a substitute for the milk or cream and butter you would usually use in the mashed potatoes. Add this puree to the mashed cauliflower and potato mixture, and this dish now gives your baby a vegetable, more protein and iron, as well as the potato. You can keep the extra puree for another time (or eat some yourself — it's good!).

Now take a look at your salad. Most salad ingredients will be a bit difficult for a baby to manage, but ingredients like cucumber can be peeled and cut into small cubes. If you have carrots in your salad, you could grate some for your baby's portion.

And what about dessert? Ice cream is not suitable for babies, and you might notice in looking at the menu that your baby has not been offered any fruit during this meal. Think about what you could include to fill this gap. Do you have strawberries in the fridge or freezer, for example? Frozen berries or peaches can be quickly thawed in the microwave. (Microwaves can heat unevenly, so stir the fruit and check for any hot spots before serving it.)

But what if your family meal includes something that isn't at all appropriate for your baby and is difficult to adapt? Either you can prepare some different items for your child's meal or keep some extra foods on hand to add to her meal to ensure the nutritional components listed previously are included.

Helpful Foods to Have on Hand

Adding these foods to supplement your family meals can help provide your baby with a healthy selection of options at every meal.

- Fresh or unsweetened frozen fruit (if you're strapped for time, consider buying pre-cut fruit that is available in many grocery stores)
- Fresh or plain (no sauce) frozen vegetables (if you're strapped for time, consider buying pre-cut veggies)
- Yogurt (unsweetened plain, or with real fruit added but no sugar)
- Hummus (plain or with mild vegetable flavors)
- Whole-grain pita or flatbreads, rice cakes or soft, whole-grain crackers (such as graham crackers)
- Cheese
- Canned beans
- Tofu
- Eggs

For example, you're eating hot dogs on white buns with french fries (something I hope you don't do too often). For your baby, you could microwave or steam some frozen broccoli florets and squash, and serve them with some canned beans that you've drained, rinsed and mashed. For dessert, you could mix a little plain yogurt with microwaved frozen blueberries and wrap it in a small piece of pita. (Or you could just plop some yogurt on top of the blueberries and let the baby go at it with her hands.) All of this will really only take a few minutes and it's much more nutritionally sound.

Remember, too, that portions should be small. Don't expect your baby to be eating more than a few bites of each food at first (although some do). You don't need to cook large amounts of food to put some aside for your baby (although, depending on your routine, you may find it's useful to make extra to save for future meals).

 Iron

The Canadian Paediatric Society recommends that foods high in iron be introduced soon after the baby starts solid foods. Iron is important for the normal development of the baby's brain and for providing the baby with the energy he needs to be active.

Babies are normally born with iron stored in their systems that will last about six months. However, some babies may experience low iron from the outset. For example, if the baby's mother didn't get enough iron before and during her pregnancy, her baby's iron stores may be lower than normal (one reason that a midwife or doctor will check the mother's iron level throughout pregnancy and may recommend supplements). As well, babies who were born prematurely and those who had a low birth weight may also not have enough iron, according to research.

A practice that can cause low iron is the immediate clamping of the umbilical cord after the baby is born. If the cord is cut quickly, the baby will get less blood transferred from the placenta (the blood flows back to the placenta) than if the cord is allowed to stop pulsating before being cut. Research has found that when cord-cutting is delayed, the risk of anemia is much lower. A 2017 study by Kc, Rana and other researchers found that waiting three minutes to cut the umbilical cord, as opposed to cutting the cord within the first minute after birth, significantly reduced the risk of low iron and anemia for babies at 8 months and 1 year. That's a long-lasting difference for just two minutes more of waiting.

Human milk does not have a lot of iron, but it is in a form that is easily absorbed. In fact, a 2009 review of six studies from around the world found that even in developing countries (where many adults have low iron), anemia was very rare in exclusively breastfed babies.

Babies on iron-fortified formula will get more iron, so giving them iron-rich solids is less of a concern. However, it's important to note that the extra iron in formula can encourage the growth of undesirable bacteria in the baby's gut, increasing the risk of gastrointestinal infections, diarrhea and constipation. These risks can heighten even more if the baby gets a lot iron from solids, too.

Generally, a low level of iron is unlikely to be an issue at this stage of your baby's life, unless he has some of the risk factors described earlier in this section. As he gets older, though, a baby who is not getting enough iron may seem lethargic, pale and have little appetite. If you notice these symptoms or have concerns, contact your doctor about testing your baby's iron level. If necessary, he can be given iron supplements (usually in the form of drops).

High-Iron Foods

- Well-cooked red meats, such as beef, lamb and venison

- Cooked lentils, chickpeas and beans

- Dark green leafy vegetables, such as spinach and broccoli

- Cooked egg yolks

It's important to note that iron from plant-based foods, such as pulses and dark green leafy vegetables, is more easily absorbed if the high-iron food is served with a food containing vitamin C. (Animal-based high-iron foods contain a type of iron that is easily absorbed without a vitamin C supplement.) Another way you can add more iron is to cook your family's food in cast-iron pots and pans.

Protein

Proteins, the building blocks of the body, are provided by many solid foods, such as meats, eggs, dairy, tofu, beans, nuts and seeds. They are also present in smaller amounts in grains and vegetables. Your baby is, of course, still getting protein from breast milk or formula as well.

Preparation • Babies with no teeth do best with ground meat that is cooked in broth (or microwaved) and either mixed with a grated vegetable or starchy food to make rough meatballs or simply put on the plate for the baby to scoop up. The baby can also be given strips of tender stewed or grilled meat big enough to grasp. Even though she can't bite off a piece, the baby can suck and gum on the piece of meat, getting lots of the juices (which contain iron) from it.

Meat with a bone in it, such as a chicken drumstick or pork chop, gives the baby a natural handle to hang onto while munching away (or sucking) on the meat. For the pork chop, you'll want to cut away most of the meat, but leave enough on the bone so that the baby can get some of the flavor and juices. Once your baby gets a few teeth, she'll be able to actually gnaw off some of the meat.

Remember, too, that meat isn't the only source of protein or iron. You can give her mashed cooked beans (and the mashing reduces the risk of the baby choking), lentils or small pieces of scrambled eggs, and these foods are easy for babies without teeth to manage. Nut butters can be spread on small pieces of bread or mixed with grated apple or mashed berries.

Healthy Fats

Fats are essential for babies and toddlers to promote brain development and healthy growth. That's why, for example, whole-fat milk is recommended for toddlers that are drinking cow's milk. It's important to understand, though, that some fats are healthier than others.

The least healthy fats are the trans fats, found most often in processed foods, such as commercially manufactured pastries and fried foods. There is no nutritional benefit for your baby to have trans fats, so if you purchase processed foods check the label to be sure it is trans-fat free. The saturated fats found in meats, dairy, some fish and eggs are also considered less healthy.

Healthier fats (which are called monounsaturated and polyunsaturated fats) are those from plants, such as nuts, seeds and some fruits and vege-

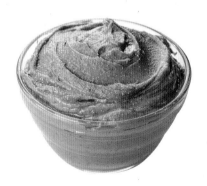

tables. Avocados are a great source of monounsaturated fat. Olive oil, another source, can be used in making mini muffins and breads. Sources of polyunsaturated fat include ground flaxseeds and ground chia seeds, which can be mixed into other foods. Some fish, such as salmon, also contain this healthier fat. Flake cooked salmon into pieces that your baby can pick up (and make sure there are no bones).

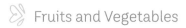
Fruits and vegetables should be the foundation of any diet. Both provide vitamins and minerals that are essential to health, as well as fiber and healthy fats. They are protective against cancers and other illnesses.

When it comes to enjoying fruits and vegetables from the outset, breast-fed babies have the advantage, as long as their breastfeeding mother eats a good variety of these foods. The flavors of the various fruits and veggies come through in the breast milk and make these foods familiar to the baby and, thus, are more likely to be accepted. A 2016 study by Maier-Noth, Schaal and other researchers found that previously breastfed children had a greater acceptance of vegetables even at age 6. They also found that introducing plenty of vegetables early on helped formula-fed babies develop a taste for them, even if they rejected them repeatedly at first.

Offering your baby a variety of fruits and vegetables is important — each fruit and vegetable contains different amounts of vitamins and minerals as well as other nutritional components in small amounts that are important for health. One way to help make sure your baby is getting a good variety is to remember the phrase "Eat the rainbow." This means offering a selection of foods of different colors — red, orange/yellow, green, blue/purple and white. Each color variation indicates the presence of different nutrients — plus your baby will probably be interested in and attracted to various hues.

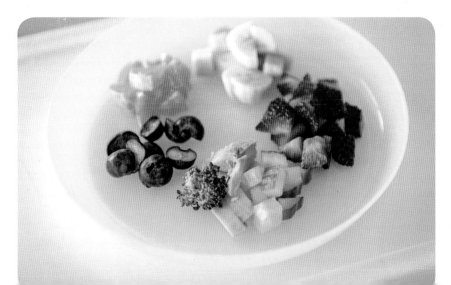

Eat the Rainbow!

- **Red** — Raspberries, red peppers, strawberries, watermelon
- **Orange/yellow** — Butternut squash, carrots, oranges, peaches, sweet potato
- **Green** — Avocado, broccoli, cucumber, kiwis, peas, spinach
- **Blue/purple** — Blueberries, blackberries, eggplant, plums
- **White** — Bananas, cauliflower, mushrooms, parsnips, potatoes

Preparation • Many fruits are soft enough for babies to enjoy as is, such as ripe pears, bananas, peaches, avocados and mangoes. Just cut them into strips (like thick french fries) so that your baby can hold them easily. Older babies who have developed a good pincer grip can pick up smaller cubes.

Firmer fruits, such as apples, can be cooked to make them easier for a baby to eat, but many babies do enjoy chomping on raw apple. To serve it, you can shred the apple with a grater or in a food processor.

Applesauce (or other pureed fruits) can be used as a dip for the finger foods the baby is eating. At first, you can dip the strips into the puree and then set them down on the plate for your baby to pick up, but in time he'll want to do his own dipping. He might also stick his fingers in the puree and lick them.

Some vegetables are good as is, such as English cucumbers, but others will be easier for your baby to manage if you can steam them until they are soft and then cool them to room temperature. Cauliflower and broccoli come in florets with a useful handle the baby can grab while gnawing on the thicker part of the floret.

Another great way to prepare vegetables is to roast them. This brings out their natural sweetness, while making them soft enough for your baby to eat easily. You can fill up an entire cookie sheet of veggies, roast them all and then keep them in the fridge to be portioned out for your baby's meals.

Once again, "Eat the rainbow" is the phrase to keep in mind here: a green vegetable, an orange/yellow vegetable and a red or blue/purple fruit will help create a healthier meal.

Baby-Led Weaning on the Go

What about those times when you're in a rush or you're planning a long drive and need to grab something from the grocery store that your baby can munch when you stop?

At times like these, it's very tempting to turn to that aisle of baby foods. You may think of grabbing some of those pouches of pureed food for convenience. Of course, nothing terrible will happen if your baby has one of those pouches occasionally, but if given too often they can divert from the lessons of baby-led weaning. The baby that is handed a pouch of pureed food has no idea what she's eating — maybe last time it was applesauce and this time it's a mixture of vegetables and quinoa. She can't make a choice based on what she wants to eat since she doesn't even know what she's getting until she sucks down the first mouthful. As well, solid foods are meant to be chewed. Digestion at this age begins in the mouth, with the digestive enzymes in her saliva, so these pureed foods will likely be less well digested when they hit the baby's gut.

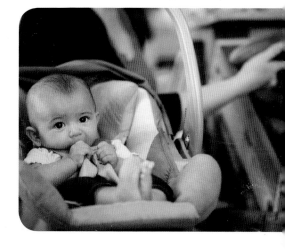

What might you offer instead? Walk over to the produce department and check out your options.

Grocery stores often sell small containers of peeled and cubed fruit that might be perfect if you cut the pieces smaller. Watermelon and mango are good options that are often available. A peeled banana cut into fingers also works well.

Does the grocery store have a salad bar or deli counter? Many of the items will be oversalted or spicy, but you might be able to find things like grilled tofu, grilled chicken, cooked asparagus spears or sliced cucumber that would work well if you cut them into smaller pieces.

For an older baby, you can look for whole-grain pita bread that you could spread peanut butter on or top with soft cheese and mashed banana and break into manageable pieces. Pretty soon you'll be used to looking around the grocery store with new eyes and seeing convenient foods for your baby in places other than the baby-food aisle.

⧉→ Drinks

Drink up! Once your baby is eating solids fairly reliably, you may start to wonder if it's time to give your baby other drinks as well. In fact, that's a good idea.

What drinks to add? The first (and best) choice is water. Plain water.

Breast milk has a perfect balance of liquids and solids that can be readily digested without putting any strain on a baby's digestive system. It also adjusts to compensate for situations in which the baby might need more liquid, such as unusually hot weather. But once you start adding significant amounts of solid foods to your baby's diet, it's helpful to also offer more liquids to make it easier for your baby to digest his food. Not enough liquid can mean he becomes constipated, his urine becomes concentrated and dark yellow or that his kidneys get overworked.

Formula puts more strain on a baby's kidneys in the digestive process. Formula-fed babies are likely to need additional water in hot weather or if they become constipated. They'll also benefit from having more water as they start solids.

Bottles and Cups

How will you give it? If you've been using bottles (either exclusively or as a supplement to breastfeeding) you might want to give water in a bottle. If not, there's really no need to introduce one to give your baby a drink of water.

There are several cup options: you can use a regular, open cup and hold it for your baby so he can sip water from it. This can be messy, and babies will often grab for the cup (making it even messier). But if you put just a little water in at a time, a cup can work well.

You can use a sippy cup, which is a lidded cup that has a small spout or opening. The baby can hold the cup without spilling too much, and if he puts the opening or spout to his mouth and tips the cup, he'll get water. Babies who have been bottle-fed usually do okay with these types of cups, although they can be a bit messy, too. Breastfed babies sometimes have trouble figuring them out, since they are not used to the flow of liquid that they get from tipping the cup.

You can use a cup with an attached straw. (A separate straw can be a choking hazard if the baby sucks it into his throat.) Breastfed babies tend to prefer these because they only get liquid when they actually suck on the straw (which is more like the way breastfeeding works). You can try it with a bottle-fed baby, too, although it might take him longer to catch on to how they work. These cups are usually less messy because the liquid doesn't pour out as easily.

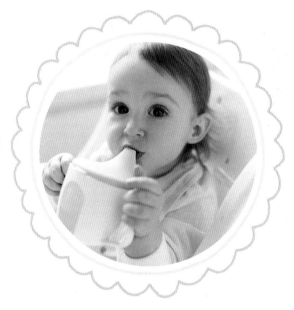

Water's good, but you may also be thinking about adding other milks (besides human milk or formula) to your baby's diet. When should you introduce them, and what are the options?

Breastfed Babies • The Canadian Paediatric Society recommends that breastfeeding continues for two years and beyond, for as long as both mother and baby choose. If you do add cow's milk (or milk alternatives, such as soy milk) after your baby starts solids, it's valuable to limit the amount so that breastfeeding can continue. You may find it helpful to give the alternate milk in a cup, so that the baby still gets his sucking needs met at the breast (which will help motivate him to keep nursing).

Formula-Fed Babies • Parents who have been paying high prices for cans of formula are often eager to switch to plain cow's milk (or other animal or plant milks) as soon as they can. You can offer plain cow's milk or dairy

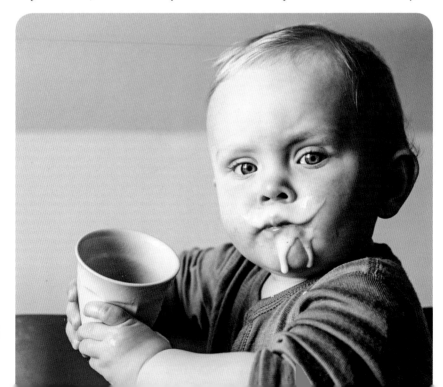

products such as cheese at any time once your baby starts solid foods, but it's recommended that formula continues to be provided until your baby is at least 1 year old and eating a good variety of solid foods. That's because there are nutrients provided by formula (including iron) that are not contained in plain cow's milk.

For vegan babies, fortified soy milk is recommended rather than other plant-based milks because it is higher in protein and calories. If you do offer, for example, almond milk rather than soy milk, make sure your baby also has plenty of other foods that are high in protein.

⤳ Taking Care of Teeth

Now that your baby is eating solid foods, you need to be thinking about wiping (and later, brushing) your baby's teeth. The age range for the eruption of a baby's first tooth is pretty wide: some babies are born with teeth, some get them in the first few months and some don't have any until after their first birthday. The average age is around 6 or 7 months, but your child may be considerably earlier or later.

Breastfed Babies

Breastfeeding mothers don't need to worry about wiping or brushing teeth and gums as long as the baby is exclusively breastfeeding. Research has shown that human milk alone does not cause cavities; in fact, it seems to help heal any gaps in the enamel. However, once a baby is eating solid foods, the mixture of human milk and solids, especially starchy or sweet foods, does put the baby at risk for cavities.

This can be a concern if your baby is nursing one or more times during the night (which most breastfed babies will be doing at 6 to 12 months). The key to reducing cavities is to clean your baby's teeth by wiping thoroughly after her last solid-food meal of the day. With no solid foods to

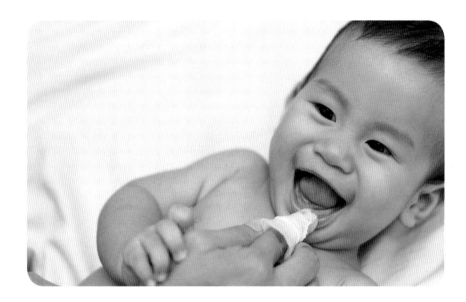

trigger cavities, your baby can then nurse at night as needed. Cleaning the teeth again after breakfast or lunch means it's fine to nurse the baby to sleep for a nap.

To clean your baby's teeth, wrap a clean, textured cloth (such as muslin) over your finger and use it to wipe your child's teeth — outside, inside and across the chewing surface. (If you are starting this early and your baby doesn't have teeth yet, just wipe her gums.)

Formula-Fed Babies

If your baby is getting formula, either exclusively or as a supplement to breast milk, keeping his teeth clean should be part of your daily routine as soon as his teeth appear. In fact, some people recommend starting this earlier so that the baby becomes used to the process and accepts it. To begin, wrap a clean, textured cloth (such as muslin) over your finger and use it to wipe the baby's teeth — outside, inside and across the chewing surface. (If you are starting this early and your baby doesn't have teeth yet, just wipe his gums.) If you don't want to clean his teeth after every feeding, ideal times to do this are after breakfast and before he goes to sleep.

⊱→ Inside the Diaper

If you've exclusively breastfed your baby prior to starting solids, you may have noticed his poopy diapers don't smell bad. That's about to change as solid foods start moving through his digestive system.

Many foods are not well-digested at first. The baby is getting some nutrients, but the more fibrous parts of the foods are going to appear in the diaper more or less the way they went into baby's mouth. Give your baby some corn, for example, and you'll probably see whole kernels appearing in his diaper. This is normal and not a big concern.

Some babies will become constipated once they get going on solids — more liquids, such as water, may help with this problem. Constipation is more likely to be an issue if you are offering your little one low-fiber foods, such as processed cereals or potatoes. Commercial infant cereals are not only low in fiber, they also contain added iron, which adds to the constipating effect. If you are using these cereals (perhaps baked into pancakes or muffins), you might want to serve them with fruit, vegetables or beans to increase the fiber.

Some babies with sensitive stomachs may develop diarrhea or loose stools. If you can trace this to a particular food, you might want to avoid that item for a few days and see if your baby's poop goes back to normal. If the reaction is severe, contact your doctor. Diarrhea can also be a sign of infection — which becomes more likely once the baby has started solid foods — so it's important to keep an eye on your baby. If he develops a fever, vomits or becomes lethargic, if his urine turns dark yellow or if the diarrhea persists for more than 36 hours, contact your doctor right away.

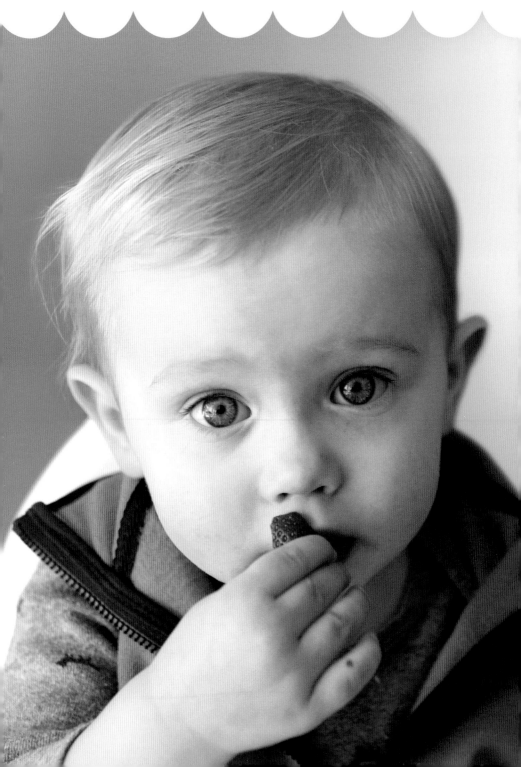

5

Special Diets

Does your family follow a special diet for ethical or health reasons? Is it important to you that your baby also follow this way of eating? If you have significant restrictions on what you eat, a consultation with a registered dietitian is recommended. This stage of life is extremely important in terms of brain growth and development, in addition to physical growth, so ensuring that your baby gets all the nutrients she needs is critical.

In this chapter you'll learn about a few of the most popular special diets — vegan, vegetarian and paleo — and explore how you might plan your baby's meals to fit your family's eating style.

⊱→ The Vegan Baby

What does vegan mean?

Vegans don't eat meat, fish, eggs or milk — nothing that was once part of an animal or comes from an animal. Some vegans do eat honey, but most do not. Many vegans also avoid animal products (such as leather or wool) when buying clothing, footwear and other products.

Of all the mainstream special diets, veganism will get the most raised eyebrows from family, friends and even some doctors if parents choose this diet for their children. While there have been cases of vegan babies who have gotten seriously ill or died because of inadequate nutrition, parents shouldn't be discouraged from raising their kids vegan as long as they're aware of what their children need nutritionally for normal growth and development.

Dreena Burton is a vegan cookbook author and a mom of three "weegan" girls. She used a baby-led approach to starting solids with her daughters and found it worked very well. "My naturopath gave us a schedule for starting solids that we modified for our plant-based diet," says Burton. "In short, we introduced certain fruits and veggies first, followed by gluten-free grains and more fruit and veg, then legumes and grains [with gluten] as well as seeds, wheat and peanuts."

People questioned her about the appropriateness of vegan eating for babies. She and her husband had already been vegan for about five years when they had their first child, and some asked whether they were going to raise their children vegan, too. "I thought that was interesting because I chose a vegan diet for myself after researching and experiencing the health benefits of eating this way. Of course I would want to give our children those same health benefits!"

While Burton's family and friends eventually understood this was a life choice, not a phase — in fact, one of her friends, along with her three children, later became vegan — she did face opposition from some health professionals. "There were a couple of times after doctor visits that I had a good cry in the car on the drive home. That was difficult, because intellectually and spiritually I knew I was doing the right thing — but when a health professional asks challenging questions, it is almost impossible not to feel emotional. I didn't have any support with an online community or other vegan parenting groups or mentors at the time. So every time I felt insecure, I would revisit my research."

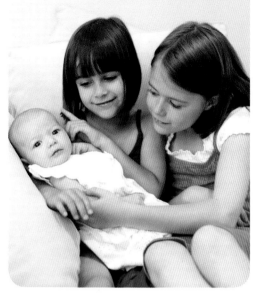

Her girls ate the whole foods that she and her husband ate. Burton recalls that her daughters' favorite foods when they were infants included sweet potatoes, peas, homemade pancakes, beans, corn, cooked pasta, pieces of tofu, fruits (like melons, berries and bananas), potatoes and home-made baked goods.

Burton worried at times that her toddlers weren't eating enough "dense" or "heavy" foods. "They just loved fruits and for some time would always [choose] fruit over breads or pasta or potatoes, or calorically dense foods like nut butters." Since the girls were active and healthy and her doctor was happy with their growth, she didn't press them to change their eating habits. As they got older, they added more of the other foods.

For Burton, one positive outcome of their vegan diet was that she never had any concerns about constipation. "In fact, I was surprised at how often they pooped! Many of my friends really struggled with constipation with their young children who were eating meat and dairy, but it was never an issue for us," Burton says. Today, she feels that raising her children vegan is one of the greatest gifts she and her husband have given them.

Being vegan is not without its dietary challenges, and parents of vegan babies may have some specific concerns about nutrition, namely, ensuring their children get enough vitamin B12, iron, zinc, protein and fats.

Getting Vitamin B12

Vitamin B12, which is essential for brain development and other vital functions, is not found in vegan foods (unless they are fortified with it, as some brands of nutritional yeast are). If the baby is being breastfed, he will get enough B12 as long as the breastfeeding mother's levels are good. Once solid foods start to significantly replace breast milk (typically at around 9 or 10 months, depending on the baby), a source of B12 is essential. If you are giving your baby soy formula, vitamin B12 is normally included in the formula.

If you are relying on fortified foods and on the amount your baby gets from breast milk, you should talk to your doctor about having the baby's blood levels tested. Vitamin B12 is essential — babies have died because they were not getting enough. It's important to have a plan to make sure this nutrient is included in your baby's diet.

There are several ways to give your baby B12: injections, sprays, fortified foods, vitamin strips that dissolve in the baby's mouth or vitamin pills (one type dissolves in the mouth and a different type can be crushed and added to the baby's food). Which is the best for your vegan baby? You may have to try more than one approach and see what works. Some are more costly than others — the spray, for example, is much more expensive than the pills.

Does giving the baby a spray, a vitamin strip or a pill violate the principles of baby-led weaning? If you feel strongly that the baby should be able to make decisions about what he eats or doesn't eat, and he's not choosing the fast-dissolving B12 pill you put on his plate, perhaps getting the injections would work better for you and your baby. Maybe let him watch you take your pill and then see if he picks up his.

There is no need to worry about your baby getting too much B12 as his body will just flush out the extra.

Getting Iron and Zinc

Even though vegans don't eat red meat or liver (the foods most people associate with iron), research has found that vegans are no more likely to be iron-deficient than those who eat meat. Iron can be found in many foods, especially in dark green leafy vegetables (such as spinach, kale and bok choy), legumes (such as lentils, black beans and soybeans) and whole grains (such as oatmeal and cream of wheat).

Iron from plants is a bit harder for the body to absorb than iron from meats, but you can increase the amount that your baby's body absorbs by serving high-iron foods with something that contains vitamin C. You don't need to add a lot — just drizzling some orange or lemon juice on top will help. If you're concerned that your baby's iron is low, you can bake and offer your baby squares or mini muffins made with iron-fortified infant cereals or cook with cast-iron pans.

Zinc is another mineral that is harder to get when not eating animal-sourced foods, but it is generally found in the same foods that have iron in them. So if you are offering your baby plenty of iron-containing foods, you're probably providing plenty of zinc as well.

Vegan-Friendly Sources of Zinc

- Wild rice and whole grains
- Cooked lentils and beans
- Tempeh
- Nuts and nut butters

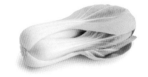

While the levels of iron in human milk are fairly low, the iron is very readily absorbed. If you have opted for soy formula, it should be fortified with zinc and iron.

Getting Protein

Got Calcium?

Many people think of calcium as something that comes from dairy products, but some of the best sources are actually plant based. Almond butter, kale, bok choy and tofu are a few good vegan sources of calcium.

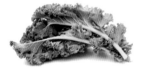

Most vegans are tired of being asked where they get their protein. Parents who are raising vegan babies feel much the same way.

Many foods contain protein. There is protein in grains and vegetables and substantial amounts in vegan-friendly foods, such as tofu, tempeh, seitan, beans, lentils, nuts, nut butters, seeds, quinoa and wheat. It's fairly straightforward to incorporate most of these into the meals you offer your baby. Tofu, for example, is an easy texture for babies to manage and will absorb the flavor of any sauce that it's cooked in. You can crumble extra-firm tofu with your fingers if you think it's too firm for your baby. Mashed cooked beans are easy for a baby to pick up (and the mashing also reduces the risk of the baby choking). Seitan can be cooked in little nuggets that the baby can pick up and chew.

Getting Enough Fats

It's important for babies to get enough fats in their diet to promote brain development and normal growth during this stage. If you're focused on keeping your diet low in fat, you may need to make modifications to the foods you offer your baby. Some options for healthy, higher-fat foods include avocado, coconut milk, nut and seed butters and vegan cheese. It's a good idea to include one or more of these in every meal you offer your baby.

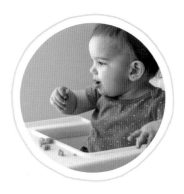

What a Vegan Baby Might Eat

One of the goals of baby-led weaning is to offer your baby healthy, whole foods that your family is eating — with some suitable baby-friendly modifications, of course. The table below shows examples of nutritionally complete meals at different stages of a vegan baby's growth — starting from 7 months, when a baby is more likely to eat whole meals.

From 7 to 9 months old	Steamed or baked sweet potato
	Steamed broccoli florets
	Mashed cooked beans and sesame seeds formed into little balls
	Slices of mango dipped in orange juice
From 9 to 12 months old	Steamed edamame beans
	Steamed green beans
	Vegan "meatballs" made with ground walnuts, vegetables and wheat gluten
	Strawberries cut into cubes
Over 1 year old	Whole-grain pita spread with vegan cheese and grated carrot
	Roasted cauliflower seasoned with curry powder
	Homemade orange-oatmeal muffin (a source of iron)

⇢ The Vegetarian Baby

> ## What does vegetarian mean?
> Vegetarians don't eat meat or fish. They do eat milk, eggs and honey.

 ## Getting Vitamin B12

Vitamin B12 is essential for brain development and other vital functions. Because vegetarians eat dairy products and eggs, they don't need to be as concerned about getting enough B12 as vegans do. If the baby is being breastfed, she will get enough B12 as long as the breastfeeding mother's levels are good.

After a vegetarian baby starts solids, if dairy products and eggs form only a very small part of the baby's diet, supplementation is possible. There are several way to give your baby B12: injections, sprays, fortified foods, vitamin strips that dissolve in the baby's mouth or vitamin pills (one type dissolves in the mouth and a different type can be crushed and added to the baby's food). Which is the best for your vegetarian baby? You may have to try more than one approach and see what works. Some are more costly than others — the spray, for example, is much more expensive than the pills.

Does giving the baby a spray, a vitamin strip or a pill violate the principles of baby-led weaning? If you feel strongly that the baby should be able to make decisions about what she eats or doesn't eat, and she's not choosing the fast-dissolving B12 pill you put on her plate, perhaps getting the injections would work better for you and your baby.

There is no need to worry about your baby getting too much B12 as her body will just flush out the extra.

Getting Iron

Parents can offer dark green leafy vegetables (such as spinach, kale and bok choy), legumes (such as lentils, black beans and soybeans) and grains (such as oatmeal and cream of wheat). Serve these foods with citrus fruits (or other foods high in vitamin C) to increase iron absorption. If necessary, iron supplements can be provided.

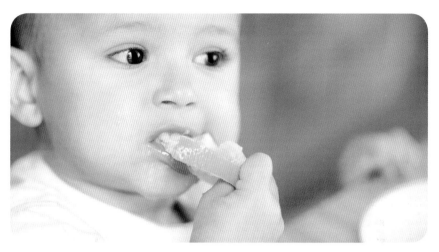

Getting Enough Fats

While adults often focus on low-fat or skim milk and low-fat dairy products, babies and toddlers should be given full-fat milk and cheese. The extra fat is important for brain development and healthy growth. Babies also benefit from getting healthy fats from nuts, grains, olives and avocados.

Too Much of a Good Thing?

It's important to be aware of the risks of overdoing dairy intake. Babies may fill up on cow's milk and cheese — which have low amounts of iron — as their main sources of protein and end up iron deficient as a result.

What a Vegetarian Baby Might Eat

One of the goals of baby-led solids is to offer your baby healthy, whole foods that your family is eating — with some suitable baby-friendly modifications, of course. The table below shows examples of nutritionally complete meals at different stages of a vegetarian baby's growth — starting from 7 months, when a baby is more likely to eat whole meals.

From 7 to 9 months old	Cooked egg yolk
	Steamed green beans
	Steamed or baked sweet potato
	Orange segments
From 9 to 12 months old	Grilled cheese sandwich made with whole-grain bread and cut into bite-size pieces
	Steamed and mashed carrots
	Sliced cucumber
	Strawberries cut into cubes
Over 1 year old	Lentil pâté spread on soft, whole-grain crackers
	Steamed broccoli florets
	Peeled kiwi cut into cubes

⤳ The Paleo Baby

What does paleo mean?

There are a few different definitions of this approach to eating, but generally "paleos" don't eat grains, dairy products (milk and cheese), legumes (beans and lentils), potatoes, sugar, processed foods or refined vegetable oils.

🐝 Getting Iron

Babies fed a paleo diet usually get plenty of iron, zinc and vitamin B12 (which is essential for brain development) from the meat in their diet. Beef, lamb and venison have the highest levels of iron if iron deficiency is a concern. Liver and kidneys are also high in iron.

🐝 Getting Protein

In the first year or so, babies may have some difficulty chewing and digesting enough meat to get the protein they need. They may suck on stewed meat or chew on meaty bones, but mostly they get the juices, which do contain iron and B12 but not much protein. Offering ground or shredded meat can make getting protein easier for your baby. You might also consider offering scrambled eggs, since they are easy to pick up and mash.

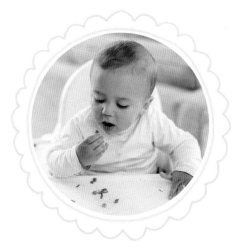

Getting Enough Calories and Fats

Another potential issue for young paleo babies is getting sufficient calories in their diet, since many of the easy, high-calorie foods — such as high-fat dairy products, potatoes and foods made with grains — are excluded, and the babies may not be eating much meat at this point. Including higher-fat foods such as avocado can help, and salad dressing can be mixed with vegetables to increase the fat level if needed. Eggs are also helpful for increasing the calories and nutrients.

Some advocates of the paleo diet suggest an 80/20 approach: they follow the diet 80 percent of the time and allow themselves to "cheat" 20 percent of the time. If this is the approach you are using, your baby's cheat foods could be easy-to-digest foods, such as grains, potatoes or beans, to increase calories.

 Constipation

Some babies (as well as some adults) experience constipation with the paleo diet if they focus more on meats and don't consume enough fruits and vegetables. If your baby becomes constipated, balance the meals by including more plant-based foods and be sure your baby is getting enough water to drink.

 What a Paleo Baby Might Eat

One of the goals of baby-led solids is to offer your baby healthy, whole foods that your family is eating — with some suitable baby-friendly modifications, of course. The table on the next page shows examples of nutritionally complete meals at different stages of a paleo baby's growth — starting from 7 months, when a baby is more likely to eat whole meals.

From 7 to 9 months old	Cooked egg yolk
	Steamed cauliflower and broccoli florets
	Orange segments
From 9 to 12 months old	Pork chop (the baby can hold the bone and gnaw on the meat)
	Mixed steamed vegetables, topped with raw avocado
	Grapes cut into quarters
Over 1 year old	Roasted cauliflower and brussels sprouts
	Chicken cut into cubes, with an orange sauce
	Slices of mango

⤳ Modifying Special Diets for Babies

Keep in mind that a baby's needs are not the same as an adult's. If you haven't chosen a special diet for health or ethical reasons, you may have adopted it because you're trying to lose weight or maintain it (most adults are). Babies, on the other hand, are growing rapidly and aiming to triple their weight in their first year. They also have an urgent need for nutrients — such as iron, zinc, vitamin B12 and fats — to support their growing brains and bodies.

Keeping that information in mind should help you make any needed modifications to your family's diet so that your baby can stay healthy. Make sure you take your baby in for regular well-baby checks. If you have any concerns or questions, speak to your doctor and ask for a referral to a registered dietitian.

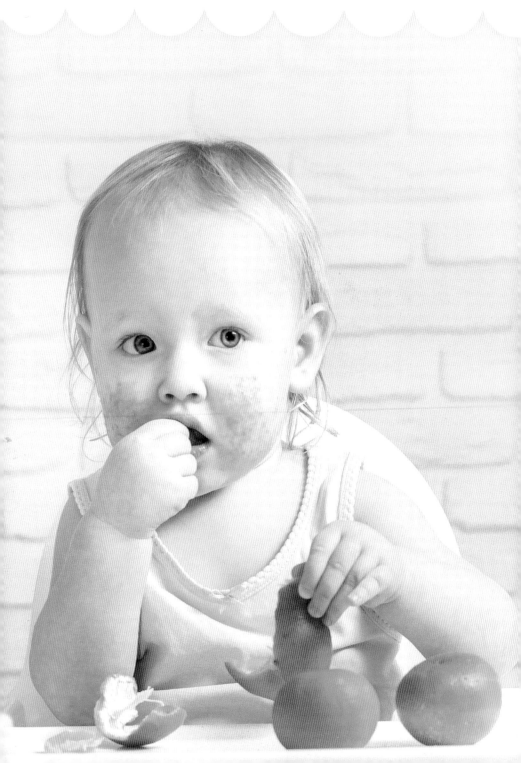

6

Allergies and Intolerances

Do you have allergies? Does your baby's other parent? While specific allergies are not inherited, a tendency to be allergic can be. With that in mind, what does a family history of allergies mean for your baby, and how might it affect your approach to starting solids?

In this chapter you will learn about some causes of allergies, possible ways to prevent them and how to approach baby-led weaning with a high-risk baby. This chapter also touches briefly on food intolerances and celiac disease.

An allergic reaction is when a person's body reacts in an intense way to a substance that is in or on the body, even though the substance is actually harmless. These reactions can range from mild to life-threatening.

When parents have a history of allergies, babies are at a higher risk of developing them. It may not be the same allergy — mom might be allergic to eggs, and baby might be allergic to cow's milk — but the tendency is what can be inherited. Parents who know their babies are at higher risk often wonder how to manage starting solids to reduce the risk of a reaction while potentially lowering the odds of future allergies.

Allergies are on the increase in North America. The Centers for Disease Control and Prevention in the U.S. reported that food allergies in children increased by 50 percent between 1997 and 2011 and now affect 1 in 13 children.

High-Risk Foods

About 90 percent of allergic reactions are caused by eight foods.

- Tree nuts (such as almonds, cashews, walnuts, etc.)
- Peanuts
- Eggs
- Cow's milk
- Soy
- Wheat
- Fish
- Shellfish

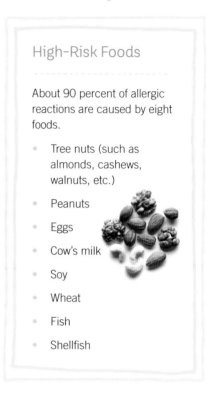

 ## Causes

What's causing this increase in allergies? There are several theories.

Hygiene

The emphasis on killing germs by using antibacterial cleansers and scrupulous cleaning means that babies and young children are exposed to fewer germs, so their immune systems have less to respond to. The immune system is geared up to battle germs, so with nothing to do, it can overreact to other new proteins that come into the body — such as food, pollutants, pollen and so on. This theory is somewhat supported by research that shows that children raised in homes with pets or on farms have fewer allergies — the idea is that the animals bring in more germs for the child's immune system to attack.

Medications

Certain medications have been linked to higher risks of allergies. A 2017 study by Ahmadizar, Vijverberg and others, and a 2016 study by Batool, Reece and others both found that the use of antibiotics in children increased the risk of developing allergies later in life. Similar conclusions have been drawn by Henderson, Shaheen and others about acetaminophen (the active ingredient in Tylenol) and by DeMuth and Stecenko about drugs that reduce acid reflux. All of these medications are prescribed and used much more frequently today than in the past.

Climate change

The warmer weather increases the length of time that certain plants release pollen into the air that sensitive children are more likely to react to. Environmental chemicals may also be an issue. For example, in a 2015 study, Sbihi, Allen and other researchers found that infants exposed to high

> ### Signs of an Allergic Reaction
>
> - Hives
> - Swelling of lips and tongue
> - Rash around mouth and/or on cheeks
> - Wheezing
> - Vomiting
> - Stomach pain

levels of car exhaust during their first year were significantly more likely to have allergies. As well, periods of smog and temperature inversions that hold pollutants close to the ground have become more common.

⤳ Approaches to Allergy Prevention

Allergies can be serious — even life-threatening — and since the percentage of children with food allergies seems to be increasing, researchers have been looking for ways to prevent them from developing. The recommended strategies have changed over the years as new research has uncovered more information.

⥈ Breastfeeding

Researchers have looked at how infant feeding can affect allergies, and their thinking about this has changed over the past decade. It's long been known, through several research studies, that breastfed babies are less likely to develop allergies. One possible reason is that breastfed babies are significantly less likely to be sick and require antibiotics, thanks to the immune factors and antibodies they receive from their mothers' milk as well as the components that nourish healthy bacteria in their digestive systems. As we know, antibiotics are linked to a higher risk of allergies.

Another suggested explanation is that, through breastfeeding, babies are exposed to small amounts of potential allergens in a way that doesn't trigger a reaction, but does teach the body that these substances are safe. Some researchers have found that when breastfeeding mothers ate peanuts, for example, their babies were less likely to develop peanut allergies. Because most parents eat a variety of foods, the baby is protected by this safe exposure to many possible allergens. Of course, this is not foolproof. Sometimes a baby will react to an allergen that comes through her mother's milk.

A 2017 study by the University of Manchester looked at infants fed human milk or formula and how the introduction of solid foods affected the subsequent development of food allergies. They came to two conclusions: the early introduction of solid foods (before 17 weeks) led to much higher rates of allergies (more than double), regardless of whether the baby was breastfed or formula-fed. However, continued breastfeeding after solid foods were introduced was associated with a lower risk of allergies. This is because certain components of human milk help the immune system recognize these potential allergens as food instead and reduce the odds of a reaction.

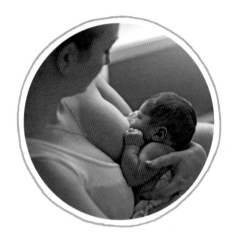

Timing Solid Foods

Studies, such as the 2017 one mentioned above, have found that very early solids (before 4 months) were clearly linked to higher rates of allergies for both breastfed and formula-fed babies. Researchers have long been interested in how adjusting this timing might affect allergy development. In 2000, based on a review of then-current research, the American Academy of Pediatrics released a statement recommending that when families have a history of allergies, parents should avoid giving cow's milk until the child is 12 months old, eggs until the child is 24 months old and peanuts, tree nuts and fish until the child is 36 months old. This statement was reviewed in 2006 and the recommendations were reaffirmed. Many parents followed this advice.

Between 2006 and 2008, however, new research appeared. A 2008 study by Du Toit, Katz and other researchers compared Jewish children living in the UK with those living in Israel. In Israel, peanuts and peanut butter were given to babies before they turned 1 (usually beginning at about 8 months)

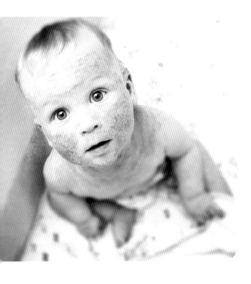

and were offered often, while in the UK, peanuts and peanut butter were typically not given until after babies were 1 year old. Ten times as many children in the UK had peanut allergies as those in Israel. Another study found that babies given eggs at around 6 months were less likely to have an egg allergy than those given eggs after 1 year. So, was the advice to wait before giving allergenic foods all wrong?

Inspired by these studies, the Learning Early About Peanut allergy (LEAP) study compared at-risk babies who were given peanuts between 4 months and 11 months (the average age of first starting peanuts was 7 months) with those who started peanuts at some point after age 1. The group that started peanuts later was six times more likely to develop peanut allergies.

Here's one theory why this might be: babies can become sensitized to peanuts by getting peanut butter or peanut oil on their skin, especially if they have eczema. But if they eat peanuts before this sensitivity occurs, the digestive system helps the baby's body to recognize peanuts as food and tolerate them rather than reacting as if they were allergens. The goal is to have the baby ingest the peanuts before the skin contact causes his body to become sensitized.

Take note, however, that eczema can also be a sign that the baby is allergic to something — either a food or something else in the environment (cat dander, for example). If your baby has eczema, it is worth being cautious when introducing solid foods.

✑→ Baby-Led Weaning for High-Risk Babies

What does this information mean in terms of starting solid foods for a potentially allergic baby?

Although some allergists have suggested starting solid foods early to introduce high-risk foods, there is no need to rush to start solids. According to the LEAP study (and most others), starting solids at around 6 months and introducing high-risk foods soon after seems to be the most helpful approach. While the LEAP study included babies who started solids as early as 4 months, the range for lower allergy rates went all the way up to babies who were introduced to those foods at 11 months, and the average age was around 7 months. So the research doesn't support pushing your baby to eat at 4 months in order to give him the high-risk foods. You can wait until he's ready.

Further, it seems that bringing these common allergens into the high-risk baby's diet fairly soon after solids are started — and offering them frequently — is probably a good idea. The average age in the study that led to lower allergy rates was 7 months, but some babies were around 11 months and still did well.

Last, for high-risk babies it's best to offer foods one at a time.

> ## Sibling Allergies
>
> Babies with an older sibling who has a peanut allergy should be seen by an allergist before being given peanuts, as their peanut allergy risk is seven times higher than that of other babies.

In non-allergic families, it's fine to mix foods up a bit, but for a high-risk baby, you'll want to start each food on its own and keep an eye out for any symptoms. That way you'll know the likely cause if your baby does have a reaction, and you can discuss with your doctor a plan to deal with it. If the reaction is severe, you'll want to avoid the food and any related foods. For example, if your child has a severe reaction to almonds, you'll want to avoid other tree nuts.

This approach can feel like a very slow start to getting a variety of foods. Let's say on day 1 you offer your baby some baked sweet potato. He likes it and — no reaction! But sometimes reactions can be delayed, so you offer sweet potato again the next day and the day after that. He still hasn't had a reaction, so day 4 can be a new food, perhaps a slice of ripe peach. Again, you keep offering peach for two more days to confirm that the baby is doing fine, and now he's ready for food number three. Nearly a week has gone by, and your baby has tried a grand total of two foods.

You can speed up the process a bit. Remember the box earlier that lists the foods that cause 90 percent of allergic reactions? Conversely, there are some foods that rarely cause allergic reactions. These other foods — for example, most vegetables and fruits, as well as most meats (other than fish and shellfish) — could be offered on one day and then something else could be added the next day. If sweet potato (which is already unlikely to be an allergen) is fine, you could probably try peach the next day and then something else on the day after that.

While it's true that some people are very specific in terms of what they are allergic to, in most cases, if you are not allergic to one food in a food family, you're probably not allergic to any of them. If lobster is fine for you, crab and shrimp probably are too.

Introducing Potentially Allergenic Foods

It's generally recommended that you start with foods that are not likely to cause an allergic reaction, because you want eating to be a positive experience for your child. If one of the first things your baby eats causes an unpleasant or scary response from her body, this could create an aversion or anxiety around eating that may affect the child for some time. It's better to have a few weeks of safer foods before you introduce any higher-risk ones.

You should also be mindful of the time and place you first offer a high-risk food. For example, when you first offer your baby peanut butter, try to do it in the morning on a day when you'll be home and be able to observe her. That's because sometimes reactions can be delayed for a few hours, and you want to keep an eye on things. If you're apprehensive, perhaps because your family has a history of severe reactions, talk to your doctor about doing this in a hospital setting.

Keep on Feeding

Once you have introduced a high-risk food with no reaction, you need to keep offering it. Otherwise, there is a higher risk of an allergy developing when the child finally does encounter it again. How often? Probably two to three times a week is enough, and the amounts do not need to be large — a teaspoon or two of peanut butter, for example, is plenty.

If your baby is not fond of the food, you might need to disguise it to encourage him to eat it. You could spread peanut butter on a slice of banana, place another slice on top and then cut the banana into small pieces for the baby to pick up. Or you could bake peanut butter into a batch of mini muffins. A high-risk food, such as eggs, could be scrambled with some meat and vegetables or incorporated into a muffin batter.

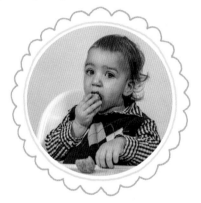

Allergy Testing

Why not just test for allergies? The problem is that these tests are not very accurate for infants — a baby can get a positive test and not be allergic or get a negative test and yet be allergic. The only truly reliable allergy test is the oral food challenge, where the baby is given the food in a safe environment. That's kind of what you are trying to do by offering these potentially allergenic foods one at a time.

If your baby has an allergic reaction, you should see your family doctor, who will refer to you to an allergist. The allergist will help you understand how to care for your baby and prevent future serious reactions. You may be prescribed medications (such as epinephrine injections) for your baby, given tips on avoiding cross-contamination or given a schedule for future testing to monitor the allergy.

⚡ Intolerances

Some of the negative reactions people have to food are not allergies — these are usually called sensitivities or intolerances. Allergies occur when the body's immune system reacts to a harmless substance in or on the body, whereas intolerances occur when the body has difficulty digesting a particular food. With intolerances, the body's reaction is typically not as dangerous as an allergic reaction can potentially be.

A common intolerance in adults is lactose intolerance, which is caused by the digestive system's inability to break down the sugar in milk. It's extremely rare in babies (although some may develop it temporarily after being ill with diarrhea), but it's common in adults. Milk is the normal food for babies, so babies produce the enzymes to break down lactose. As some young children get older, they stop producing these enzymes. For those adults, drinking cow's milk (or eating dairy products such as cheese) can cause stomach cramps and diarrhea.

In some parts of the world, especially in Europe, cows (and other animals) have been raised for food for thousands of years. As well as eating the animals, people also drank the cow's milk. As this practice spread, the proportion of people who produced the enzymes to digest cow's milk increased.

Even if you or your partner have problems with lactose intolerance, though, it is very unlikely that it will affect your baby.

Celiac Disease and Gluten Intolerance

Gluten is a protein found in wheat, barley, rye and other grains from the same families, as well as grains that might have wheat in them as a result of accidental mixing. Some gluten-free diets are stricter than others. People with celiac disease, a serious autoimmune disorder, have to be very careful to avoid all gluten and foods that could be contaminated with gluten, but those who are less sensitive may be able to eat other grains.

Celiac disease affects a person's intestines so that any gluten — even very small amounts — will cause the intestinal lining to inflame, which leads to intense pain, bloating and diarrhea. Those who are celiac must be very careful with their diet. For example, a piece of gluten-free bread toasted in a toaster recently used for a slice of wheat bread could be contaminated enough to make the person seriously ill. Celiac disease is genetic, so your baby's risk is higher if you or a relative have the disease.

Sometimes a baby will be diagnosed as celiac, but in other cases the diagnosis is not made until the child is older. Current testing requires the baby to be exposed to gluten, so testing and diagnosis can't really be done until the baby starts solid foods. If the baby is celiac, parents will have to be careful to avoid other grains that might have become contaminated, such as oats, unless they are certified gluten free.

Other people are gluten or wheat intolerant. While these people do not have celiac disease, eating foods with gluten in them or eating wheat upsets their digestive system and causes bloating, gas and pain.

Many gluten-free products are available in stores, but often these have a lot of added sugar and salt, so they are not suitable for babies. There are now basic gluten-free flours that you can use at home to bake for your baby.

> To learn more about foods containing gluten, visit:
> celiac.org/live-gluten-free/glutenfreediet/sources-of-gluten/

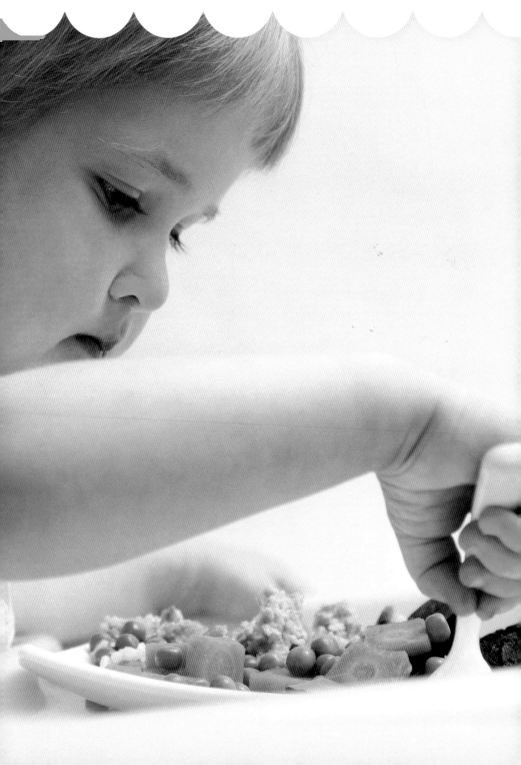

7

Continuing On with Healthy Eating

Baby-led weaning has given your baby a great start. He's learned to respond to his own internal cues about eating, enjoy health-promoting foods and enjoy the social aspect of mealtimes. Now you want to keep that going — not always easy in a world of fast-food restaurants and snacks with cartoon characters on the box.

In this chapter we'll offer some ideas for busy parents about how to continue the healthy eating path they've started.

⤳ The Division of Responsibilities Rule

Dietitian Ellyn Satter has outlined a very helpful rule for parents:

> Your job is to provide and offer healthy foods; your child's job is to decide what and how much to eat.

It's a great statement to remember. Just as it was when your baby was first starting solids, your responsibility is to keep offering appropriate foods for your child to choose from.

Satter's rule is also very important to remember when you find yourself arguing with your child about eating. In those situations, are you trying to take over your child's job? Maybe it's time to step back.

⤳ Introducing Utensils

Baby-led weaning involves a lot of finger foods, but as your baby grows into a toddler, you will want to introduce the idea of using a spoon and, later, a fork. There's no particular age when you should do this; your baby will probably let you know when she wants to try it out. Choose a toddler-sized spoon — wood or plastic is easier on baby's teeth if they get banged, and they might!

The easiest first step is to use a pre-loaded spoon. Use something that is thick enough to stay on the spoon even if it gets waved around a bit, such as hummus, nut butter, mashed potato or a semi-solid pureed soup. Put a little on the spoon, enough to give the child a good taste, and then set the spoon down on her usual tray, with the handle pointing toward her. If your baby is already looking at the spoon with interest, it's fine to help put the spoon in her hand. You're probably going to have to load up the spoon for quite some time, because it takes babies time to develop the coordination to dip a spoon into a semi-liquid food and transport that food to their mouths.

Some parents will help the toddler if he's getting frustrated — once he's shown that he wants a spoonful of the soup or other food item, they'll spoon it into his mouth for him. Though you're technically spoon-feeding, this is still considered a baby-led approach. Again, it's important to follow your baby's cues. If he loses interest after two or three spoonfuls, it's time to stop. Ali's son, Walter, who's almost 2, will tap the side of his bowl of soup to indicate that he would like a spoonful. She'll give him one or two spoonfuls, and then he might pick up a slice of cucumber and take a few bites before tapping on the bowl again. "He's very clear about what he wants," Ali says.

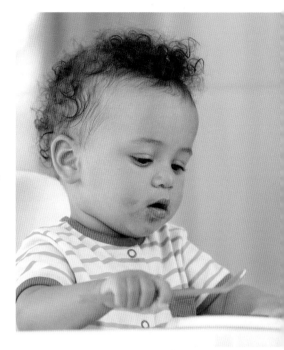

As time goes on, though, your toddler will be able to start using a spoon more effectively.

There's no rush to introduce a fork, but in time your baby will be able to use it to pick up pieces of thicker food, such as braised meats or grilled tofu. A metal fork is preferable — even though there is the risk of her poking herself or you or the dog with it. But by the time she's ready to use a fork, she will have a bit more control. Plastic and wooden forks are too frustrating and flimsy for a toddler to use.

Your toddler might also be interested in using a knife because she sees you using it. If she's past the age of flinging utensils around, a dull, metal butter knife should be fine. She will most likely just imitate what she sees you doing: trying to cut with it or using it to spread toppings on bread or crackers.

ᗘᐳ Understanding Appetite Ups and Downs

During the first five or so months, the average baby will double his birth weight, and by 1 year he will have tripled his birth weight. That's why young babies feed so often. But after the first year, the rate of weight gain slows down significantly. The average weight gain between the first and second birthdays is 5 pounds (2.3 kg); for some toddlers it's as little as 2 pounds (0.9 kg) and a few will gain a bit more than average. Five pounds is about 20 percent of the weight of an average 1-year-old, so this is a *much* slower rate of weight gain than the 300 percent gain expected in the first year.

As a result, toddlers tend to have smaller appetites than when they were babies, and this often worries parents. The child who enthusiastically gobbled down a plateful of food even after a full breastfeeding or bottle of formula is now only willing to eat a small portion at each meal. Multiple research studies, including a 2014 study by Birch and Doub, have shown that pressuring toddlers to eat doesn't improve their eating. It is, however, linked to later eating disorders, as found in a 2015 study by Matheson, Camacho and others.

This is a good time to remind yourself of the Ellyn Satter rule. Your job: preparing and serving healthy foods. Your child's job: deciding what and how much to eat. Yes, it can be frustrating to prepare a meal and set it out for your toddler only to have him pick at it, maybe eating one or two mouthfuls and then ignoring the rest. But attempts to persuade him to eat are more likely to backfire than be productive. You particularly want to avoid mealtime battles when you say things like, "You'll sit there until you eat it all!"

It can help to offer the more reluctant eater just a little bit of food at a time. Shelley, a mother of three, found that her toddler seemed to be overwhelmed when she put a full plate of food on the table in front of him. "It was like he was afraid that if he got started he'd have to eat the whole thing," she says. "So he'd rather eat nothing at all." She switched to a smaller plate that was divided into sections and put just a small portion of each food item in each section. "That made a big difference. And if he ate it all and was still hungry, I had no problem giving him seconds."

As long as you make the food available, your child will take what he needs. Learning to listen to his body and respond to his body's signals is a very important part of his development.

It's also frustrating for parents that toddler appetites can vary quite drastically. One day, your toddler might eat a lot, the next day, very little. Or you may have several days of enthusiastic eating, followed by a week of eating almost nothing. As annoying as this is, it's perfectly normal. Some days your child is growing more than others, and some days he is more active than others (and therefore using up more calories). Even something like learning a new skill can use up a lot of energy and create a bigger appetite. On the other hand, stressful experiences can reduce an appetite.

All these fluctuations are to be expected. If you can deal with them calmly — for instance, just taking away the plate once your toddler's lost interest or dinnertime is over — your toddler will develop the healthy eating habits you'd like him to have. That doesn't mean giving him a time limit, like "Eat this in the next 15 minutes or I'm taking your plate away." It means that when everyone else is done, you pick up your toddler's full plate as you clear the table. Of course, if he then protests and says, "Don't take that away, I want more," you can give it back.

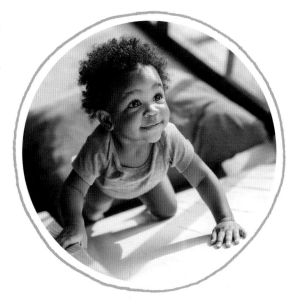

ᴥ→ Building Good Eating Habits

Remember your job: you are in charge of deciding what foods you serve your child. So if you want your child to eat health-promoting foods, such as fruits, vegetables, beans and whole grains, then that's what you put on the plate. It will help if you eat those foods yourself, because children want to imitate their parents. (The food on your plate always looks better to them, even if you're both eating the exact same thing.)

Your baby's food preferences are set in these early years. It's those foods you remember from childhood that make you feel happy, secure and loved during the tough times in life — what we think of as comfort foods. These

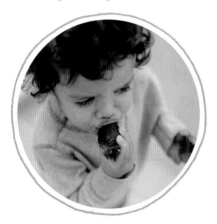

are the flavors and textures that will be familiar and that your child will be drawn to as she grows up. Not only that, but feeding your child well now sets a foundation of health. This is a time of rapid brain development, a time to create strong, dense bones and a time when the gut microbiome is maturing. Focus on healthy foods to give your child a healthy beginning.

What's the Gut Microbiome?

"Microbiome" is the word used to describe the collection of microorganisms that live in a particular environment, such as the intestines (or gut) of a person. Each of us has a large number of bacteria, fungi and viruses living inside us. When everything is in balance, the bacteria and other microorganisms help us digest food and stay healthy in ways that we are really just starting to understand.

Foods to Offer

As you did when your baby was starting solids, ensure that you offer a variety of foods that cover all the nutritional needs of your growing toddler. Ideally each plate should include the following:

- Fruits and vegetables. Try to make them easy to eat and appealing (which may mean steaming, roasting, peeling the stalks or cutting the food into slices or interesting shapes)

- An iron-rich food: meat, egg yolks, lentils, beans, chickpeas, leafy green vegetables

- A source of vitamin C to increase iron absorption, especially for plant-based sources of iron: orange, grapefruit, strawberries, kiwi, mango

- A source of protein: tofu, beans, lentils, cheese, yogurt, meat, fish

- A source of healthy fats: nut butters, seed butters, avocado, fish

- Whole grains prepared so that a child can easily eat them: oatmeal, whole wheat breads, brown rice, quinoa

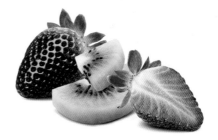

Start to introduce foods with a variety of flavors. Foods with mild spices and flavors such as garlic and ginger will encourage your toddler to enjoy more food options and not expect only sweet, salty or fatty foods.

Foods to Avoid

To help build good eating habits and keep your toddler safe, you will want to avoid the following foods, if you can:

- Foods that increase the risk of choking: grapes, hot dogs, raw carrots, nuts, hard candies, popcorn

- Honey (for babies under 1 year because of the risk of botulism)

- Fried foods: chicken nuggets, french fries, doughnuts

- Foods with added sugars: cookies, ice cream, candy

- Salty foods: potato chips, pretzels, other snacks

- Processed meats of any kind, since these contain chemicals linked to cancer and may be contaminated with bacteria linked to serious infections

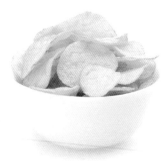

- Sugary drinks: fruit juices, soda pop, sports drinks

Nothing terrible will happen if your child eats less-healthy options once in a while, and it's not necessary for them to have every nutrient every day. However, the sweet/salty/fatty flavors can become addictive for many kids. They have plenty of time to discover these foods.

If your schedule or situation means you have to eat at fast-food restaurants, you have some options. You can pack food to bring with you for your baby or toddler. Many fast-food restaurants have healthier things on the menu, or, if there are no healthy options, you can try to make modifications. For example, if the only menu option for your little one is chicken nuggets, peel off the fatty coating on the outside before offering them. See if you can order a baked potato or apple slices instead of french fries — these are options at some fast-food places now. To make things like the baked potato or apple slices small enough for your toddler to manage, you can bite them into smaller pieces, use a plastic knife at the restaurant or bring a paring knife with you for cutting. Keep in mind when your child won't have any vegetables at a meal and consider offering some when you get home.

⊱→ Dealing with Picky Eaters

If you've followed the advice of exclusively breastfeeding for six months and starting solids after that, you've already taken a big step toward preventing picky eating, according to the 2011 Synergistic Theory and Research on Obesity and Nutrition Group Kids (STRONG Kids) study by Shim, Kim and others. The researchers found that children who started solids before

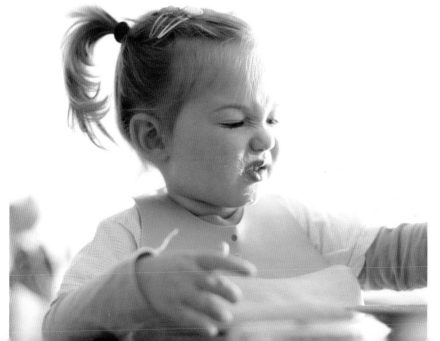

6 months were 2.5 times more likely to avoid new foods and eat only a limited variety of foods. Exclusively breastfeeding until 6 months reduced the risk of these behaviors by about 80 percent.

But of course, that's not a guarantee. Maybe you've done your best, but despite it all you have a child who says she hates all vegetables. You try not to give in to it, but all she wants to eat is toast and jam. Or perhaps she's willing to eat a wider variety of foods, but there are a lot of rules: the foods can't touch each other on the plate, or everything has to be cut into the right number of pieces. The appearance of a new food on the plate is greeted with great suspicion, and no, she is not going to take a bite. Now what?

There's a school of thought that says these picky behaviors might have evolutionary benefits. In this world, where some foods might be poisonous, caution about new foods can be a good thing. The berries from *this* bush might be safe, but the berries from that bush could make you very sick. This caution about food tends to arise just at the age when toddlers are getting more independent and might get into things they shouldn't be eating, so the tendency might well be protective.

All the same, it drives parents crazy. The solution? Just keep offering. Don't put much of the new food on her plate, since she probably isn't going to eat it, but keep right on offering. One study found that, on average, a new food had to be offered 12 times before a child would eat it, but once the child tried the food, most of the time that food became acceptable and was readily eaten after that. What seems to happen is that as the food keeps reappearing on the plate, it becomes familiar. Something that looked gross and unappealing before becomes "Oh, that again" to your toddler. Familiar foods are safe and more likely to be accepted.

There are other possible causes of picky eating. Some children have strong gag reflexes that can be triggered by foods with certain textures. Anything that is hard to chew, has strings (like celery) or is persistently lumpy can set off the gag reflex and cause the child to reject the food. You might be able to solve part of this problem with different methods of preparing and cooking foods.

Some children have food sensitivities that are not actually allergies, but that can leave them with digestive problems. They may turn down those foods without being able to explain why. It can be important to respect this, as that food may be a health issue for the child.

What about the kind of pickiness that says food has to be cut into quarters and arranged on the plate so that nothing touches? Or the child who will only drink his milk from the blue cup with Mickey Mouse on it? To a certain extent, that's just toddlers being toddlers. They are seeking more control in their lives, and this is another area in which they can try to do it. Try to be calm and matter-of-fact about these demands. If you can reasonably comply (cutting a piece of toast into four pieces is no big deal), then go along with it. But if, for example, the blue cup is in the dishwasher and it's almost time to go to work, you just may have to say, "You can have the milk in one of these three cups, but those are the only choices."

If you find yourself trying to piece together a cookie that accidentally broke because your child will only eat a whole cookie, you're trying too hard. He may need to have a good cry over the broken cookie, but that's okay.

Strategies for Picky Eaters

- Stay relaxed and calm if your child rejects a food. Getting annoyed or angry won't help.

- Continue offering foods that your child has rejected without putting pressure on her.

- Eat as a family as much as possible so your child can see others enjoying the food she has been reluctant to try.

- Don't praise, reward or make a big fuss when your child does try the food. Her mealtimes shouldn't be about making you happy.

If your child's aversion to new foods stretches into the preschool years, these steps can help him to explore new foods in different ways. Instead of asking him to eat the food, ask him to go through as many of these steps as he's comfortable with.

1. Look at the food. Ask your child to describe it.

2. Touch the food. Ask for a description of what it feels like.

3. Taste the food by licking it or touching it to the tongue to get a brief taste. Ask what it tastes like and whether it reminds your child of any other foods.

4. Take a bite.

You may not get to step 4 until you've done the first three steps over a period of several days. If the process works well, you could ask if he'd like to take two bites next time.

Constipation and Diarrhea

Constipation is a major concern for many parents of toddlers. A study by Yong and Beattie found that 36 percent of toddlers were constipated, and another study found that 58 percent were constipated by that study's definition — two or fewer bowel movements per week and stools that were hard when passed.

A 2011 study by Afzal and Tighe also found about half of the preschoolers they followed were constipated. The main causes they identified were as follows:

- They were not getting enough fiber.

- They consumed too much milk or dairy products.

- They did not consume enough water or other liquids.

So if your toddler is constipated, what can you do? First, try to drop or at least significantly reduce some of the low-fiber foods that may be creating the problem: anything made with white flour, dairy and meat. It can be hard to bring in higher-fiber foods if your child is filling up on higher-fat dairy and meat, which will make her feel full. These foods are good for growth, but if a child has become constipated, her diet is likely unbalanced. Then start offering more foods that have substantial amounts of fiber. Beans are an excellent source, and they come in a variety of flavors, are easily mashed to combine with other foods and have lots of protein as well. Most fruits and vegetables are good sources of fiber, too, so offer those as much as possible. Also offer plenty of water to drink.

If your child's constipation does not resolve with these diet changes, consult your doctor. Managing constipation is important because if it is not dealt with immediately, it can become an ongoing problem: the bowel can become stretched and less sensitive to the signals that say "it's time to go," and chronic constipation is not only unpleasant but also linked to other health issues.

Diarrhea in small children is most often caused by a virus, bacteria or some other infection rather than a reaction to food, although it can be a sign of food intolerance. Remember that human milk causes loose stools, and a child who is still nursing will probably continue to have soft stools even though he's getting some solids too. Some children who are eating a high-fiber diet will have frequent, fairly loose stools (two to four per day) even if they are not breastfeeding, but this should not be confused with diarrhea. True diarrhea in a toddler means watery, often explosive bowel movements very frequently throughout the day — often every hour or so. The child may show signs of dehydration (his urine is dark yellow, for example) and a fever. If the diarrhea lasts for more than 36 hours or your child becomes lethargic or is also vomiting, call your doctor.

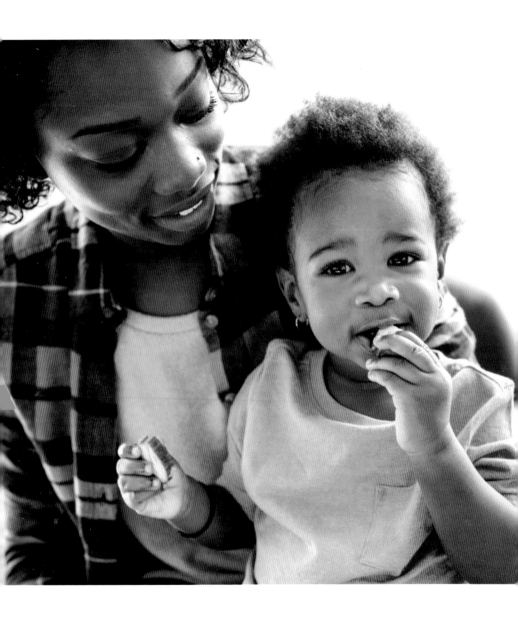

⤳ The Basis of Lifelong Healthy Eating

Baby-led weaning doesn't guarantee that your child will never steal cookies from his brother's lunch or try some fad diet to lose 10 pounds. But based on everything we know about how healthy eating patterns develop, this approach seems to offer the best foundation for future eating.

The baby who started solids this way has learned to:

- Listen to her body about what she wants to eat and how much
- Stop when she's had enough, even if there is food left
- Eat because it's what she wants, not to make someone else happy
- See mealtimes as social events, shared with her family
- Avoid foods she dislikes or that make her feel uncomfortable (which may signal an intolerance)

If you keep on reinforcing these lessons as your child grows, she'll have the best chance of continuing to eat in a healthy way.

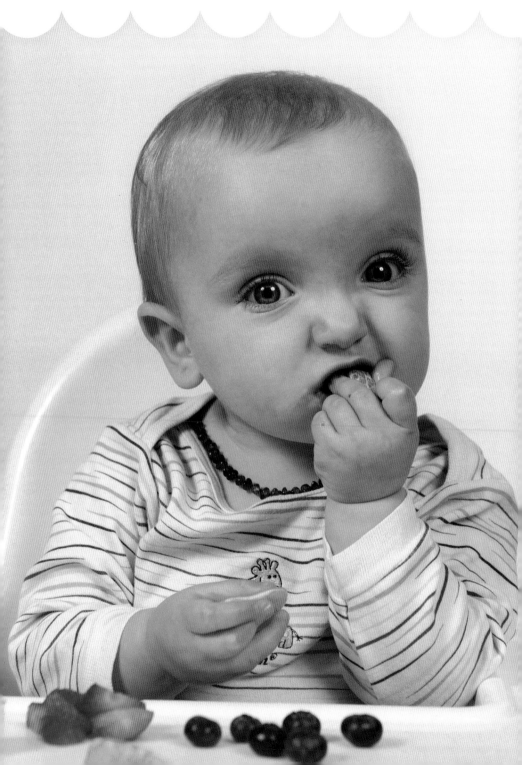

8

Frequently Asked Questions

While we've tried to give an extensive overview of baby-led weaning, you might still have questions. Here are answers to some of the more common questions parents ask about various aspects of starting solids using the baby-led approach.

⤳ About Baby-Led Weaning

You recommend starting solids at 6 months, but won't starting solid foods earlier (like at 3 or 4 months) help my baby sleep longer?

A common reason parents give for starting solid foods early is to make the baby sleep longer. If the baby is waking at night, perhaps it means he's hungry, and adding solid foods could solve that problem and get everyone more rest. We get it — lack of sleep is the bane of all new parents, and you may be willing to do pretty much anything for an extra half hour of shut-eye.

However, it's normal for babies to wake during the night for feeding. First of all, they are trying to double their weight in the first six months and triple it by the time they are 1 year old. If you were trying to double your weight, you'd probably need some midnight snacks, too.

Night feedings are especially important for breastfeeding. Prolactin, the hormone that promotes the production of human milk, is produced in larger amounts during night feedings, encouraging the breasts to continue making plenty of milk. If night feedings are dropped too early, the mother's overall milk production can decrease significantly. This is a problem especially if the mother has a low milk storage capacity. Renowned lactation expert Professor Peter Hartmann has shown through his extensive research that while almost all women can produce enough milk to meet their babies' needs over 24 hours, some women can store more in their breasts than others. The mother who can store, for example, 4 ounces (118 ml) in her breasts can feed her baby less frequently than the mother who can only store 2 ounces (59 ml). If the breastfeeding mother has a smaller storage capacity, dropping night feedings can make it very difficult for her baby to get enough milk.

Of course, there are other factors, too. Some babies have smaller stomachs than others, so even if the mother can provide 4 ounces at a feeding, the baby may not be able to comfortably drink that much. And babies nurse for reasons other than hunger — they may want the closeness, the comfort of suckling or just a drink because they are thirsty or hot.

Last, research has found that adding solid foods does not cause babies to sleep longer at night. In fact, some babies begin waking more, probably because the solids are upsetting their digestive systems. This makes sense, because many babies who eat substantial amounts of solid foods at 12 or 15 months old still wake up at night — a 2015 study by Murthy and Bharti found that 80.7 percent of toddlers wake up one to three times during the night. So solids can't be the cure-all for that issue.

My baby was born prematurely. Should I start offering solid foods when he is actually 6 months, or should I go by his "corrected age"?

The corrected age is the age the baby would have been if he'd gone to full term (which is 40 weeks). So, for example, baby Sebastian was born at 32 weeks — 8 weeks premature. At 6 months from the day of his birth, he'll be just 4 months old according to his corrected age.

Registered dietitian Jennifer House says she generally advises parents to go by the baby's corrected age. So if you were Sebastian's parents, you'd be looking for signs of readiness and offering him his first foods when he's close to 8 months old (from the day of his birth) because that's when, physically and developmentally, he's more like a full-term 6-month-old.

The big concern with a premature baby, House points out, is that he may need iron earlier than when he is ready to start eating solids. That's because babies store iron during the last weeks and months they are in utero. So a baby who is born early hasn't had enough time to get his full share of iron. (In contrast, babies who are born past their due date have the benefit of extra iron stores.) While the amount of iron stored in a full-term baby is typically enough to last six months or longer, the premature baby may only have enough to last a couple of months, so it's likely to be used up by the time he's reached his "corrected age" of 6 months.

Usually, parents of premature babies are advised to give their babies iron drops to supplement the small amount in breast milk. (If you are formula-feeding, you would give the standard iron-fortified formula.) If you have not been giving your premature baby iron, you could ask your doctor to check his iron level at 4 months or so to see how he's doing. If it's low, beginning iron drops could be an option if your baby is not ready for solids.

I started my baby on infant cereal and jars of pureed food a couple of weeks ago. I'd never heard about baby-led weaning before and that just seemed like the right thing to do. Now I'd like to switch to a baby-led approach. Can I do that? Will my baby be confused?

Of course you can! In fact, most parents who start with pureed foods or infant cereals find that as the baby gets older, she starts wanting to pick up her own food. She'll grab for the spoon, reach for the food on dad's plate or take dog food out of the bowl. You can help that process by getting rid of the pureed food and offering solid foods that she can pick up herself. Most babies her age are picking up toys, pieces of dirt and anything else they can reach. So when you put some chunks of banana or a piece of a muffin on her plate, she'll probably grab it and stick it in her mouth at some point. That's the beginning!

Some people recommend that if you have started on purees, you might want to take a break from solids for a week or so before introducing finger foods. Their concern is that because babies learn to open their mouths and swallow when given purees, they might try to do the same with solid pieces of food and end up choking. You will need to make up the calories for the waiting period with extra breast milk or formula.

If you have half-finished boxes of cereal and jars of pureed food sitting around, remember that you can use them in preparing solid foods for your baby. Infant cereals can be baked into breads, pancakes and muffins, and pureed fruits can be mixed into muffins or used as a sauce or dip. See chapter 9, pages 175–179, for some recipes that use infant cereal.

A big part of introducing solids the baby-led way is being patient and following the baby's lead. Not all babies are ready to eat other foods at 6 months, and those who are not tend to behave exactly the way you have described. They enjoy playing with their food, even exploring it with their mouths, but they are not ready to chew and swallow the food. That's okay.

Readiness for solid foods has much to do with development. Many things need to come together, some of them visible (the baby's ability to sit up and reach for food, for example) and some of them invisible (such as the development of the baby's stomach and intestines). It sounds as if your baby has the ability to sit well and grab the food, but apparently some other aspects of development haven't quite caught up.

You could try offering foods that taste sweet — like human milk — and can be mushed easily in his mouth if he does decide to chew a bit. Bananas or pieces of very ripe peach are often popular with babies at this early stage.

Try not to worry too much. He'll be ready soon enough.

Registered dietitian Jennifer House says that most babies will start solids by the time they are 8 months old if they are given frequent opportunities to try. But the truth is that some won't. As it turns out, these are most often breastfed babies, and that's good, because a baby can go longer on just human milk than on formula.

For the baby who is still rejecting food at this age or beyond, House recommends asking your doctor to test the baby's iron level. That's really the main nutrient to be concerned about. If her iron level is good and she is active and gaining weight appropriately, then you can keep on being patient a bit longer. If your daughter's iron level is low, you can give her iron supplements. As well, a low zinc level can suppress the appetite, so that's another possible nutrient to test for and supplement.

In most cases, you baby should start eating solids before 10 months. If that hasn't happened, you may want to talk further with your doctor. There are sometimes physical or developmental reasons for the delay that should be checked out.

> I feel like my baby is wasting a lot of food with the baby-led approach. He eats some, but a lot ends up on the floor or his shirt. I think it would be a lot more efficient to just spoon it in.

We all want to be more efficient in our daily lives so we can get the most work done in the least amount of time. But when it comes to a baby or child learning a new skill, efficiency is often the enemy of learning. While it's true that it's probably faster and less messy for you to feed him, you risk getting in the way of him learning to do it for himself. You'll see the same pattern as your child grows and has to master things such as cleaning his room, dressing himself, helping with the dishes, even doing his homework. You could do all these things more efficiently, but you'd be depriving him of the chance to learn for himself.

And yes, it will feel like some food is wasted, but that is part of the learning process as well. He will sometimes pick up too much and drop some as he tries to move it to his mouth — but eventually he'll figure out how much his hand can hold. He is learning about texture and consistency as he spreads the food on his high-chair tray.

It can help to put smaller amounts of food on his tray or plate and add a bit more after he's eaten the first serving. That gives him less to play with (and some babies signal that they are "all done" by throwing any leftover food onto the floor). But generally it helps to accept that the learning process is often messy and inefficient.

My toddler is 15 months old now and we've been mostly pleased with how well baby-led weaning is going. But sometimes I get frustrated by how long it takes him to eat a meal. I will put out food for him and he eats it, plays with it, babbles to me, eats a bit more, then plays around some more. It can easily take 45 minutes for him to finish! Sometimes I think he's finished so I start to take the food away, and he gets very upset and cries. Can I speed this up at all?

This is pretty common! Not all babies are like that — some are voracious and enthusiastic eaters who are very focused on their meals. But many will eat this way, adding lots of playtime and social time to their meals.

This can be a positive thing. People who are trying to manage their weight are often encouraged to eat more slowly and with others. This slower pace gives the stomach time to register how full or not full it is and signal whether more food is needed. Sometimes people end up overeating when they eat quickly, because they don't get that signal until they've already over-filled their tummy. (This can happen when you are spoon-feeding a baby.)

You might be able to focus him on his food by bringing his attention back to it when he starts to talk to you or play: "Look, a yummy piece of cauliflower! Doesn't it look delicious?" Another approach that sometimes works is putting out a small amount of food at first. Once he eats that, offer a little bit more. This reduces his playing with the food (since there's less to play with), and if you offer something different each time, he might be intrigued by the new item.

Some kids are also very easily distracted if they are eating with older siblings or other children — too much activity and excitement. For those situations, it may be better to give him a little food to play with during family meals and provide the rest of the food to eat at a quieter time.

> You should see my baby's face every time I offer her a new food! The first time she had a slice of clementine, she scrunched up her eyes and twisted her mouth — you would think I'd given her a slice of lemon. I gave her some meat, and she grimaced like it was the worst thing ever. Why is she reacting like that?

Babies have no filters. Whatever they are experiencing is going to show on their faces. Infant taste buds are also more sensitive than adult taste buds — any hint of sourness or bitterness is magnified for them. Yet it rarely discourages them from eating. I've watched babies eat slice after slice of orange, making that same "yuck, sour" face each time, but then they keep going back for more as soon as one bite is chewed up and swallowed.

Make sure to take some photos — they can be very entertaining!

> My son is like a little squirrel — he stores food in his cheeks. He just keeps putting food in his mouth and ends up with a big portion of it in his cheeks. Sometimes he spits it all back out, other times he will eat it later. Is this normal?

This is pretty common behavior, and there are two possible causes. One could be that your little guy is too eager to eat food and not very good at chewing and swallowing yet. Perhaps he gets a piece of food in his mouth, starts to chew it, notices something else he wants to eat, puts that in his mouth, too, and then pushes the first piece of food into his cheek to make room. Because he's not yet skilled enough, he might have trouble getting the food out of his cheek and back into his mouth, so eventually he spits it back out.

The other possible cause is that your son may have some difficulty with managing food in his mouth — perhaps he has tongue-tie or some other physical challenges. If he has had other feeding struggles, you might want to consult your doctor or an occupational therapist.

But otherwise, it's probably just a case of too much food at once. Try offering smaller amounts or one food at a time and then bringing out more food once the first pieces are eaten.

Every time I give my baby a plateful of food, she eats all of it. Is this normal?

You might just have a hungrier-than-average baby. However, if your baby was bottle-fed in a non-paced way, she may have gotten used to finishing the bottle every time, and this could have taught her to eat the whole plateful. You might try putting out small portions of food at meals instead. Once she has eaten her small portion, wait to see if she still seems hungry. If she is, give her a bit more. Watch again to see if she's hungry before offering more again. Over time, the goal is to teach her to pay attention to her body's signals.

⤳ About Health and Nutrition

I always put out four or five foods for my baby — trying to make sure all the nutrients are covered. But he only eats one or two things and that's it. I'm worried he isn't getting all the nutrients he needs.

When you start solids, breast milk or formula should still provide most of your baby's nutrition, so don't worry if he doesn't eat everything you offer — your milk will fill in the gaps.

As your baby gets older and solid foods become a bigger part of his diet, keep in mind that your child's body (like yours) is able to store most nutrients. Rather than looking at a single meal, or even a single day, consider his intake over the week. If he ate only fruit on Monday, did he catch up by eating more protein on Wednesday? In most cases when parents have these concerns, they find it all evens out over a few days.

If it doesn't — maybe your baby seems to only want to eat fruit, for example — you could try making some meals without his favorite food or with just a small amount of it. You might also try serving his food in stages: offer the type of food he hasn't been eating much of first, then bring out the more favored food afterward.

Another possibility is combining foods. Are grated apples a favorite but vegetables tend to get left behind? Try mixing in some grated carrot with the apple or cooking some apple and spinach together. Does he like mashed sweet potato but is ignoring protein? Mash in some beans or some drained and rinsed canned salmon.

My 7-month-old baby is enjoying eating solids, but when I change her diaper I see much of the food coming through unchanged. Is she actually getting any nutrients out of her food?

There's a saying that goes, "Food before one is just for fun." It's not completely true, but sometimes it helps parents feel more relaxed about this phase of starting solids. Your baby is still getting most of her nutrients from breast milk or formula at this age, and what she gets from solids is more supplementary.

Fruits, vegetables, legumes and whole grains all contain fiber, which is basically the part of the food that can't be digested. This is good, because fiber is important for health and digestion — not enough fiber causes constipation and intestinal gas and is linked to chronic health issues later in life. Adults chew their food well, so the fiber tends to be in smaller pieces and not as noticeable in their stools, but babies (who might not even have teeth) don't usually chew thoroughly, and so the fibrous parts pass through the digestive tract in larger pieces. The baby is still able to extract the nutrients and calories from the food as it passes through.

Even sucking on a piece of food will give the baby some nutrients. For example, if your baby sucks on a piece of cooked steak, she will certainly get some nutritional value from the juices she has consumed.

> Lunches and dinners seem pretty straightforward, but I am not sure what to give my baby for breakfast. My usual breakfast is a cup of coffee and a doughnut, and I know that's not suitable for him!

Breakfast doesn't have to be restricted to what we think of as traditional breakfast foods. There's no reason not to give a baby leftovers from yesterday's dinner or more of the kinds of things you'd offer him for lunch or dinner.

If you're looking for more traditional breakfast ideas, consider these: whole-grain toast topped with nut butter and mashed banana; whole-grain toast topped with mashed avocado; whole-grain toast topped with soft cheese or hummus; whole-grain pancakes, crepes, waffles or pita bread with similar toppings or fruit toppings; scrambled eggs or tofu with cheese and chopped vegetables; smoothies with milk, veggies, fruit or nut butter; healthy homemade mini muffins; and thick, cooled oatmeal. With older babies who have a good pincer grip, you can offer whole-grain commercial cereals (without milk) — the baby can just pick the pieces out of the bowl.

> My 10-month-old daughter seems to really like solid foods, but now she's losing interest in her bottles. She's down to about three bottles in 24 hours now, and I'm worried that's not enough. Won't she miss out on important nutrients if she isn't drinking enough formula?

Your daughter can get all the nutrients she needs from foods other than formula, as long as you are paying attention to offering her appropriate, nutritious foods. She could have some cheese, for example, to give her the protein and calcium she would get in her formula. While formula can provide enough nutrition for a young baby to grow, the added nutrition from solid foods is needed by the second half of the first year.

It's still good for her to have formula until she is 1 year old. Three 8-ounce (237 ml) bottles a day should be plenty at this stage. If you are concerned that she's not taking enough, you might replace some of the water you are giving her with formula.

You do want her to eventually wean from the bottle, so this may be a good thing!

My family — and my doctor — are concerned about my son's small size. They don't believe he is getting enough to eat from baby-led weaning.

Some children are genetically smaller than others. Has your doctor been concerned about your child's weight all along, or is this something new? You might want to talk to your doctor to hear the specific concerns.

Research has shown that baby-led weaning provides plenty of calories. However, if you do need to increase your son's caloric intake, the goal would be to offer more calorie-dense foods. Think about ways you could add fats, proteins and starches to his diet while not neglecting fruits and vegetables. If you are offering him pieces of waffle for breakfast, for example, you could spread the waffle with nut or seed butter and top it with banana and blueberries. Mash some hummus into sweet potatoes and serve it with steamed broccoli florets. Make small homemade meatballs to go with roasted brussels sprouts that are drizzled with an oil-based salad dressing.

⤳ About Eating Out

We have a family vacation coming up, and I'm concerned about my 1-year-old eating in restaurants. She is eating well, but I'm worried about what to feed her when we eat out. My mother-in-law was saying it would be better to buy her jars of baby food, but I know she won't eat purees.

Restaurants can be a challenge with toddlers no matter what approach you are using. Toddlers are usually not keen to sit for long and may not eat well because of all the distractions around them — and then they get cranky because they're still hungry.

If possible, pack some non-messy foods that you know she likes for her mealtimes, or plan to drop by some grocery stores while traveling. You might find that it's easier to eat at "fancier" restaurants than at fast-food places. Typically, fast-food places have a restricted menu, with food that's prepared in advance, so they don't have much flexibility to make foods that your baby likes and that you feel okay giving her. But a casual dining restaurant is likely to have an actual chef or cook in the kitchen and ingredients like vegetables, fruits and meats that can be turned into a toddler-appropriate dish if you ask. (The chef is more likely to be able to make something different if you drop by the restaurant at a less-busy time — say a late lunch or an early dinner.) Be sure to bring a nice big bib that covers all her clothes to help make her meal less messy (and a bag with a change of clothes is always a good idea with kids this age).

You might also want to order a meal for yourself that includes some things she might eat. Toddlers often like to eat from a parent's plate, and that seems to be more likely if you are in a restaurant. Restaurants are strange environments to toddlers, and they may feel more secure sharing a parent's food.

If it's a lively restaurant, she might not eat much at all. Don't worry about this, since you can bring food back with you, and she'll probably be happy to finish it up in the car (have someone sit beside her while she's eating) or when you get back to the hotel.

We are planning to go camping as a family this summer, and my 8-month-old is just getting good at eating. What can I bring for him to eat on our trip?

Will you have a cooler with ice or ice packs? How long will the trip be? A baby is more susceptible to the various bacteria that can grow and multiply in food that is not kept at a safe temperature. If the weather is hot, the food will start to go bad more quickly.

Look for things that can be kept for a period of time at room temperature — or warmer — and try to keep other things as cool as possible. Some options include:

- Canned vegetables and beans
- Canned fruit, such as pears, peaches, etc. (bring extra water to rinse off the sugary syrup)
- Pouches of tuna (no draining needed)
- Packaged whole-grain crackers

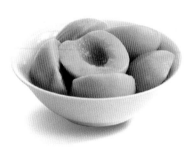

You can bake and prepare foods like pancakes or breads in advance and bring them along. They will not last as long as the canned foods, but they should be safe for the first day or two.

Your first step is to talk with the day care staff and see if this is negotiable at all. If you sent a prepared lunch, ready-to-go, would they be willing to offer it to your daughter? This will make more work for you in the morning, though, so take that into consideration. There are plates for babies that come with lids that seal tight, which might make it easier to transport and serve.

It's likely that older babies or toddlers at the day care are fed in a more baby-led way, with food put in front of them to select rather than having it spooned into their mouths. Depending on how the day care is set up, you might be able to ask whether your baby could be fed with the older ones if the staff looking after younger babies aren't willing to change their feeding routine.

If you aren't able to persuade them to switch, and don't have another day care option, you may need to let them do it their way. You can use a baby-led approach for breakfast and dinner, and on the weekends, while the staff continue to spoon-feed your daughter during her day care lunches. She'll eat most of her meals with you and will still benefit from the self-feeding skills she learns.

⤳ About Special Situations

Whether you are supplementing with a feeding tube at the breast or with a bottle (which is more common), it can be a hassle.

Dr. Jack Newman, a Toronto-based pediatrician who specializes in breastfeeding (and is the author of the foreword in this book), often suggests starting solids at around 4 months for parents in this situation. It can make continuing breastfeeding easier, and often the alternative is switching to formula or adding it, which he believes is less desirable than continuing breastfeeding and supplementing human milk with healthy, whole foods.

Yes, adding solids earlier does increase the risk of infection, but so does adding formula. Also, adding solids is preferable because breastfeeding is more likely to continue. That's because if you add formula, you are probably going to use a bottle, which can change how the baby sucks at the breast. The bottle may also seem easier for your baby because of the consistent, fast flow of milk he receives through the nipple, so in that way it can interfere with continued breastfeeding. When you offer solid foods instead (and no bottles), the baby will retain his natural need to suck and want to spend time at the breast, which helps to keep breastfeeding going.

But what if you want to introduce solids, but your baby doesn't show signs of readiness or is uninterested in solids when you offer them to him? It may be worth continuing to try. Look for foods with appealing tastes for babies (such as bananas, peaches and other soft, sweet foods) that will be easy for even a 4-month-old to pick up. When you put the food in front of your baby, have him sit on your lap so he feels secure. Offer the foods cut or cooked in different ways to see if something captures his interest.

Usually breastfeeding mothers are advised to breastfeed first and offer solid foods afterward, but if you are trying to encourage a somewhat reluctant baby to eat solids, you might want to try the opposite: offer the solids when the baby is hungry and breastfeed afterward.

If your baby is interested and begins eating solids, introducing foods that are higher in protein and fats will help you move away from supplementing as quickly as possible. Try to keep the foods healthy, though — for example, chicken nuggets do have both protein and fat, but they aren't suitable for infants.

My baby seems to have difficulties with eating in general. She had a hard time with breastfeeding as a newborn, and now she struggles with self-feeding solids. Sometimes she seems to be trying to eat a piece of food, but it ends up falling out of her mouth. I wonder if it would help if I spoon-fed her.

Before you turn to spoon-feeding your daughter, it might be a good idea to ask your doctor to refer you to an occupational therapist or another feeding expert. Some children have anatomical problems that make feeding difficult — such as a tongue-tie, which can be treated. Other children may need help mastering their feeding skills. It's good to do this as soon as you identify there is an issue because, depending where you live, there can be a long waiting list for evaluation and treatment.

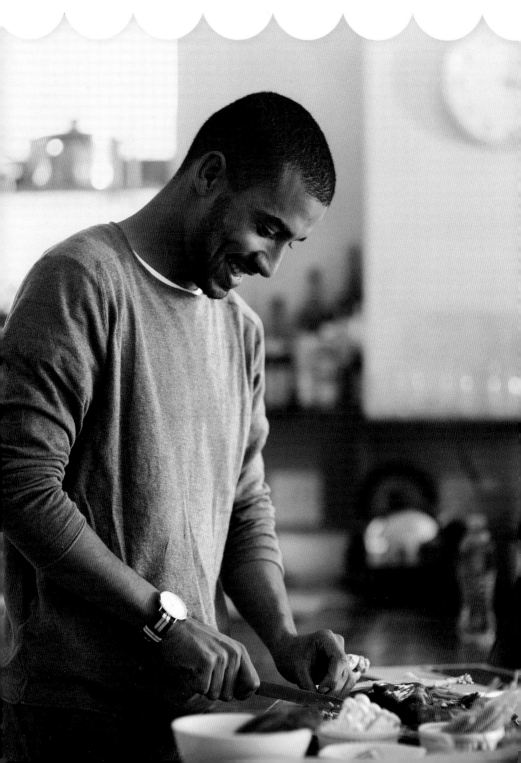

9

Baby-Friendly Recipes

One of the goals of the baby-led weaning approach is providing your baby with the foods that the rest of the family eats and enjoys. Much of the time your baby will be able to share meals with you, but it is often helpful to have some foods on hand to round out your baby's food selection when your own meal has ingredients that are not suitable for an infant or when you want to provide more choices. With that in mind, here are some simple recipes that your little one might enjoy — and that might give you ideas about more ways to prepare food for your baby. Vegan-friendly recipes have been marked with a ♥ symbol.

⤳ Recipes for 6 Months and Up

When you start solid foods, simple cooking is the best approach. Your baby is eating small portions, and often the easiest strategy is to give her a little bit of what you are eating (before adding any salt, sweeteners, sauces or spices). Here are some recipes to help round out some of those meals.

Roasted Vegetables ♥

This is an essential (and easy) recipe that you'll come back to time and time again.

Assorted vegetables cut into strips for a baby to grasp easily, about 1 inch (2–3 cm) wide, 1 inch (2–3 cm) thick and 3 to 4 inches (8–10 cm) long, depending on the vegetable

- Preheat the oven to 400°F (200°C).
- Line a cookie sheet with non-stick foil or lightly spray with non-stick cooking spray. Place the vegetables with a longer cooking time on one side of the cookie sheet and cook for 20 minutes.
- Turn the vegetables over and then add the veggies with a shorter cooking time. Cook for another 10 minutes.
- Turn over just the vegetables with the shorter cooking time, and cook for another 10 to 15 minutes. Before removing the veggies from the oven, test that they are softened and tender enough for your baby.
- Cool to room temperature before serving.

Vegetable Roasting Times

Here are some popular vegetables to roast. Sort them by length of cooking time. The precise length of cooking will depend in part on how big your pieces are, so keep an eye on them.

40 to 45 minutes: Sweet potatoes, butternut squash, potatoes, brussels sprouts and carrots

20 to 30 minutes: Bell peppers, zucchini, portobello mushrooms, green beans (with fibrous ends cut off), cauliflower florets and broccoli florets

Easy Ground Beef with Vegetables

This is a good recipe for adding iron to your baby's diet. If you cook this in a cast-iron skillet, the vitamin C in the tomatoes will help the baby get even more iron. The sweet potato is a good source of vitamin A.

½ lb. (225 g) ground beef

½ 28 oz. (825 ml) can no-salt-added diced tomatoes, drained

1 cooked sweet potato, peeled and cubed

- Slowly brown the ground beef in a pan over medium heat (this way you don't have to add oil).
- Once it is cooked through, add the diced tomatoes and cook the mixture for about 5 minutes.
- Add the cubed sweet potato and cook for another 5 minutes.
- Mash all the ingredients together toward the end, cool the mixture to room temperature and form it into little balls small enough for your baby to grasp.

Cooked Fruit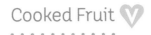

Harder fruits, like apples and pears, can be softened on the stovetop so that they're safer for babies to eat.

Apples, pears or peaches

- Cut the fruit into slices about 1 inch (2–3 cm) thick.
- Pour a little water into a cast-iron or another heavy-based pan, place the pan over medium heat and add the sliced fruit. Cover and cook until the fruit is tender (10 to 12 minutes for apples and pears, and 5 to 10 minutes for peaches).
- Cool to room temperature before serving.

Banana Treats

Many babies like the sweetness of bananas. In this recipe the wheat germ provides a source of iron, and the orange juice helps with iron absorption.

1 ripe (but not overripe) banana, cut into fingers or small chunks

Orange juice

Wheat germ

- Dip each piece of banana in orange juice and then roll it in wheat germ. You can mash the coated banana a bit if your baby prefers.

Yogurt Ice Pops

This makes a nutritious treat for hot weather.

1 cup (250 ml) plain yogurt or yogurt with unsweetened fruit

½ cup (125 ml) no-sugar-added applesauce (can be blended with other fruit)

- Mix the yogurt and applesauce well, and pour the mixture into ice pop molds.
- Freeze for 30 minutes, and insert a rounded wooden ice cream stick (make sure the sticks are food safe). Freeze the mixture for another 1 to 2 hours to be sure the ice pop is completely frozen before offering it to your baby, and keep an eye on your baby as he eats toward the stick.
- Instead, you may choose to make these in an ice cube tray and give them to your baby without the stick. Messier, but still tasty!

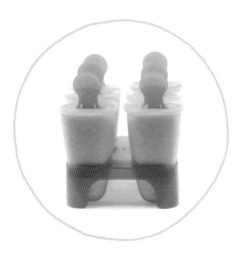

↣ Recipes for 9 Months and Up

As your baby gets older and expands his intake of solids, he'll be able to eat more of your regular family meals. These recipes will help when you want to add some extra nutrition.

Apple Pear Sauce ♥

This is a versatile snack that you can use to sweeten other early foods or as a dip. I recommend using Gala apples and Bartlett pears for this recipe.

3 apples, cored and cubed (approximately 4 cups [1 l])

3 pears, cored and cubed (approximately 3 cups [750 ml])

½ cup (125 ml) water

- Combine all of the ingredients in a medium saucepan and place over medium-low heat.
- Simmer until the apples and pears begin to break down and they fall apart when mashed with a fork.
- Let the apple and pear mixture cool, and then transfer it to a blender or food processor. Blend until smooth.

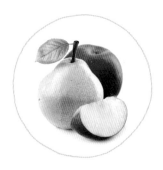

Classic Hummus ♥

This simple hummus is mild in flavor.

6 tbsp (90 ml) water

¼ cup (60 ml) tahini

3 tbsp (45 ml) fresh lemon juice

2 tbsp (30 ml) canola or olive oil

½ tsp (2 ml) sea salt

½ tsp (2 ml) cumin

1 19 oz. (540 ml) can chickpeas, drained and rinsed (or about 2 cups [500 ml] cooked chickpeas)

- In a food processor, combine all of the ingredients and blend until smooth.
- Store the hummus in an airtight container in the fridge for up to two weeks. It also freezes well.
- Hummus is good for spreading on other foods, using as a dip or pre-loading on a spoon. As your baby gets older, you can add more spices and blend in some cooked vegetables.

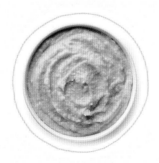

Sweet Potato Dip ♥

This dip has a wonderfully subtle sweetness that makes it a favorite with toddlers.

1 medium sweet potato, peeled, cut into chunks and steamed until soft (approximately 1 cup [250 ml])

1 19 oz. (540 ml) can chickpeas, drained and rinsed (or about 2 cups [500 ml] cooked chickpeas)

¼ cup (60 ml) tahini

¼ cup (60 ml) fresh lemon juice

1 tsp (5 ml) ground cumin

½ tsp (2 ml) sea salt

Pinch freshly ground black pepper

¼–⅓ cup (60–75 ml) water

- In a food processor, combine all the ingredients and blend until smooth, adding water as needed to create a thick, creamy consistency.
- Store the dip in an airtight container in the fridge for up to 10 days.

Socca (Chickpea Flour Pancake) ♥

Because *socca* is made with chickpea flour, it is very high in protein. *Socca* is very mild in flavor and makes a great base for a variety of toppings. This recipe is from Nicole Axworthy's blog, *A Dash of Compassion*.

1½ cups (375 ml) chickpea flour

1¾ cups (425 ml) warm water

3 tbsp (45 ml) olive oil

¾ tsp (4 ml) salt

½ tsp (2 ml) black pepper

* In a large bowl, whisk together all the ingredients and allow the mixture to sit undisturbed for 20 to 60 minutes.
* Preheat the oven to 500°F (260°C). Line two 8-inch (20 cm) round pans with parchment paper.
* Pour half of the batter into each pan.
* Bake for 5 to 8 minutes until the mixture is firm and the edges are set.
* Turn the oven setting to broil, and broil for 3 to 5 minutes, until the tops are lightly browned.
* Remove the pans from the oven. Use a knife to loosen the edges, and then flip each piece onto a plate and peel off the parchment paper.
* Let the bread cool to room temperature and then cut it into pieces as desired.

Meatloaf

· · · · · · · · ·

This recipe makes a tender meatloaf with a mild flavor. To serve the left-overs to adults or older children, you might choose to make a gravy or sauce to pour over each slice to enhance the flavor.

1½ lb. (700 g) ground beef

1 egg

1 onion, chopped

1 cup (250 ml) milk

1 cup (250 ml) quick oatmeal

Salt and pepper to taste (but minimize the amount of salt for your baby)

- Preheat the oven to 350°F (180°C).
- Mix all the ingredients together thoroughly, and pack the mixture into a 5-by-9-inch (13 x 23 cm) loaf pan.
- Bake for 1 hour. Insert an instant-read thermometer. If it reads 160°F (71°C), the meatloaf is done.
- Let the meatloaf cool to room temperature and cut it into small cubes or rectangles.

Perfect Pancakes

These perfect little pancakes contain no gluten, nuts or animal products.

1 cup (250 ml) rolled oats

½ cup (125 ml) uncooked millet

¼ cup (60 ml) coconut flour

¼ cup (60 ml) sunflower seeds (raw, no shell)

1 tbsp (15 ml) chia seeds

1 ½ tsp (7 ml) baking powder

¼ tsp (1 ml) cinnamon

2 cups (500 ml) non-dairy milk

½ tsp (2 ml) vanilla

3 tbsp (45 ml) maple syrup

Coconut oil

- In a food processor, combine the dry ingredients, and blend until the mixture has the consistency of flour.
- Add the milk, vanilla and maple syrup, and blend into a smooth batter.
- Heat a skillet over medium-low heat and lightly grease the pan with coconut oil. Allow the skillet to heat up for a few minutes.
- Pour the pancake batter into 4-inch (10 cm) circles in the skillet, and cook for 2 to 3 minutes, or until small bubbles appear on the surface and the edges look dry. Flip the pancakes and cook on the other side for about 1 minute. Transfer to a plate.
- Let the pancakes cool to room temperature, and cut them into pieces as desired.

Banana Mini Muffins

This is a tasty muffin with a small amount of sugar that is easy to take along on outings.

2 cups (500 ml) whole wheat pastry flour

½ tsp (2 ml) salt

3 tsp (15 ml) baking powder

½ cup (125 ml) sugar

¼ cup (60 ml) olive or canola oil

¾ cup (175 ml) milk (non-dairy is fine), with 1 tsp (5 ml) apple cider vinegar mixed in

3 ripe bananas, mashed well

- Preheat the oven to 350°F (180°C), and spray a 24-cup mini-muffin tin with non-stick spray.
- In a large mixing bowl, combine the flour, salt and baking powder.
- In a medium bowl, whisk together the sugar, oil, milk and vinegar mixture and mashed bananas.
- Add the wet ingredients to the dry ingredients, and stir until combined.
- Scoop the batter into the muffin tin and bake for about 15 minutes, until the edges and tops are lightly browned and an inserted cake tester comes out clean.
- Let the muffins cool to room temperature. Depending on the age of your baby, you may want to break the muffins into smaller pieces.

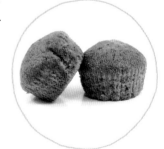

ᛦ→ Recipes for 12 Months and Up

By this age, most babies have a good mouthful of teeth, which makes it easier for them to eat a wider variety of foods. Their coordination is better, too, so they can pick up and manipulate foods they couldn't manage six months ago.

Braised Chicken Thighs

The dark meat of chicken contains more iron and is often cheaper than the white meat. Here's a simple way to prepare chicken thighs so that they're easy for a baby to eat. You can add vegetables to the oven-cooking part as well. If you have one, a cast-iron skillet makes this easier (and adds more iron). Cooking the thighs with the skin on improves the flavor and fat content.

4 chicken thighs

1 tbsp (15 ml) olive oil

½ cup (125 ml) no-salt-added chicken stock

vegetables (optional)

- Preheat the oven to 350°F (180°C).
- In a skillet, heat the olive oil over medium-high heat, and brown the chicken thighs on both sides. If you're using an ovenproof cast-iron skillet, add the chicken stock to the skillet, along with any vegetables, and put the whole thing in the oven. If you don't have a cast-iron skillet, transfer the chicken to an ovenproof casserole dish and add the stock and any vegetables to the dish.
- Bake the thighs for 40 to 45 minutes. Remove the skin before giving the chicken thighs to your baby.

Carrot Mini Muffins

. . . .

This recipe is an easy way to sneak some vegetables into your baby's diet. In place of carrots, you can use zucchini or combine half carrots and half zucchini.

2 cups (500 ml) whole wheat pastry flour

½ cup (125 ml) sugar

1 tsp (5 ml) baking soda

1 tsp (5 ml) baking powder

½ tsp (2 ml) salt

½ tsp (2 ml) cinnamon

2 medium carrots, grated

¾ cup (175 ml) milk

½ cup (125 ml) applesauce

¼ cup (60 ml) olive or canola oil

½ cup (125 ml) raisins

- Preheat the oven to 400°F (200°C), and spray a 24-cup mini-muffin tin with non-stick spray.
- In a large bowl, combine the flour, sugar, baking soda, baking powder, salt and cinnamon.
- In a medium bowl, combine the carrots, milk, applesauce and oil.
- Add the wet ingredients to the dry ingredients and stir gently until mixed. Stir in the raisins.

- Scoop the batter into the muffin tin and bake for 10 to 12 minutes, or until an inserted cake tester comes out clean.
- Let the muffins cool to room temperature. A toddler should be able to manage eating these mini muffins, but you can break them into smaller pieces if you'd like.

Black Bean Filling

This mild filling can be shaped into little balls to be baked, served in wraps or spread on bread or crackers. The filling is high in iron, protein and fiber.

1 tbsp (15 ml) olive oil

1 onion, finely chopped

2 cloves of garlic, minced

1 red pepper, finely chopped

1 tsp (5 ml) apple cider vinegar

1 19 oz. (540 ml) can black beans, drained and rinsed

- In a skillet, heat the olive oil over medium heat. Add the onion, garlic and red pepper, and cook until the pepper is soft and the onion is lightly browned.
- Add the vinegar and black beans, and mash the beans in the pan, mixing them in with the vegetables. Once the filling is well mixed, cook it for another 5 minutes.
- Let the mixture cool and use as desired.

Banana Nut-Butter Ice Cream

This is a great frozen treat with no added sugar. If your toddler is good with a spoon, she can eat it that way, or you can serve it wrapped in a crepe or in an ice-cream cone.

2 frozen ripe bananas

2 tbsp (30 ml) no-added-sugar nut butter (peanut, almond and cashew butters are all good options)

- In a food processor, combine all the ingredients and blend until smooth. Add a tablespoon (15 ml) or so of water if needed. The mixture will look lumpy at first and then will turn into a smooth and creamy treat.

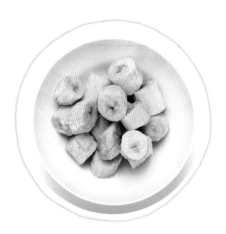

ꙮ→ Recipes Using Infant Cereal

These recipes are adapted from ones shared on the HealthLink BC website and are particularly helpful if you were given infant cereal or you want to add more iron-rich foods to your baby's diet. Infant cereal has iron added to it, so these foods can all be considered good sources of iron.

Oatmeal Pancakes

· · · · · · · · · · · · · · · · · ·

These pancakes make a healthy, high-iron breakfast. You can add berries or chopped fruit to the batter or as a topping.

²/₃ cup (150 ml) rolled oats

1½ cups (375 ml) water

2 eggs

3 tbsp (45 ml) canola oil

½ cup (125 ml) whole wheat flour

1 cup (250 ml) infant cereal (any variety)

2 tbsp (30 ml) sugar

1 tbsp (15 ml) baking powder

Olive oil

- Mix the rolled oats and water in a bowl, and let the mixture soak for 5 minutes. Mix in the eggs and canola oil, and stir until well combined.
- In a larger bowl, combine the flour, infant cereal, sugar and baking powder.

- Add the wet ingredients and mix thoroughly. The batter should be fairly smooth, but slightly mushier than usual pancake batter.
- Heat a skillet over medium heat and brush it with olive oil. Pour 2 tablespoons (30 ml) of batter in the skillet and cook for 2 to 3 minutes, or until small bubbles form on the surface and the edges look dry. Flip the pancakes and cook on the other side for 1 minute.
- Let the pancakes cool to room temperature and cut them into pieces, as desired.

Infant Cereal Mini Muffins

These high-iron muffins are easy for a toddler to eat and can be broken into smaller pieces for a younger baby. You can also add fruit such as blueberries or chopped dates if you'd like.

1 cup (250 ml) whole wheat flour

½ cup (125 ml) sugar

2 tsp (10 ml) baking powder

1 cup (250 ml) infant cereal (any variety)

½ cup (125 ml) water

2 tbsp (30 ml) olive or canola oil

3 eggs, beaten

- Preheat the oven to 350°F (180°C), and spray a 24-cup mini-muffin tin with non-stick spray.

- In a bowl, combine the water, oil and eggs.
- In another bowl, combine the flour, sugar, baking powder and infant cereal.
- Add the wet ingredients to the dry ingredients and mix well.
- Scoop the batter into the muffin tin and bake for about 15 to 20 minutes, or until an inserted cake tester comes out clean.
- Let the muffins cool to room temperature. Depending on the age of your baby, you may want to break the muffins into smaller pieces.

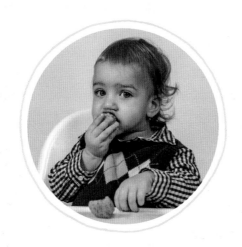

Molasses Biscuits

· · · · · · · · · · · · · · · · · ·

Molasses is a source of iron, so combining that sweet flavor with infant cereal makes these biscuits an even better source of this essential nutrient.

¼ cup (60 ml) molasses

¼ cup (60 ml) butter or non-hydrogenated margarine, room temperature

1 egg

1 tsp (5 ml) vanilla

¾ cup (175 ml) whole wheat flour

½ tsp (2 ml) baking soda

2 cups (500 ml) infant cereal (any variety)

3 tbsp (45 ml) water

2 tsp (10 ml) cinnamon (optional)

- Preheat the oven to 350°F (180°C).
- In a bowl, mix the flour, baking soda and infant cereal.
- In a larger bowl, combine the molasses and softened butter or margarine. Stir in the egg and vanilla.
- Pour the dry ingredients into the wet ingredients. Add the water and cinnamon (if using) and mix thoroughly, until you have a dough.
- Pinch off walnut-sized pieces of dough and roll the pieces between your hands to make small balls. Place the balls on a lightly greased cookie sheet and bake for 10 to 12 minutes.
- Let the biscuits cool to room temperature and break them into smaller pieces for your baby, if needed.

Oatmeal Biscuits

· · · · · · · · · · · · · · · · ·

These biscuits are milder in flavor than the molasses biscuits, but they still offer a good amount of iron for your growing baby.

2 cups (500 ml) rolled oats

¼ cup (60 ml) whole wheat flour

1 cup (250 ml) infant cereal (any variety)

2 tsp (10 ml) baking powder

1 tsp (5 ml) cinnamon (optional)

½ cup (125 ml) butter or non-hydrogenated margarine, room temperature

½ cup (125 ml) brown sugar

2 eggs, beaten

- Preheat the oven to 350°F (180°C).
- In a bowl, mix the oats, flour, infant cereal, baking powder and cinnamon (if using).
- In a larger bowl, mix the softened butter or margarine with the sugar and eggs.
- When they are thoroughly combined, add the dry ingredients and mix well, until you have a dough.
- Pinch off walnut-sized pieces of dough, and roll the pieces between your hands to make small balls. Place the balls on a lightly greased cookie sheet and bake for 10 to 12 minutes.
- Let the biscuits cool to room temperature and break them into smaller pieces for your baby, if needed.

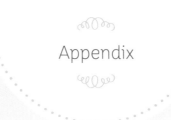

Appendix

Baby-Led Weaning in Practice

Babies all over are already experiencing the benefits of baby-led weaning! These photos, submitted to us by enthusiastic parents from the Facebook group Baby-Led Weaning (BLW) Canada and others, show babies and toddlers who are discovering food and learning about their bodies.

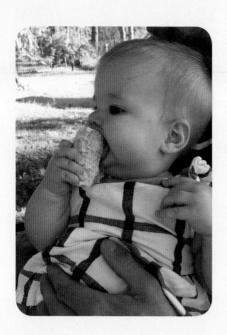

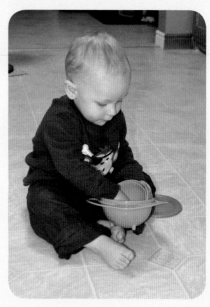

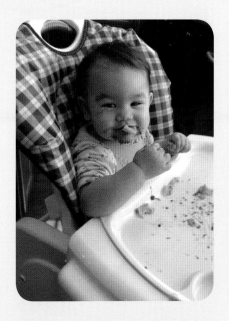
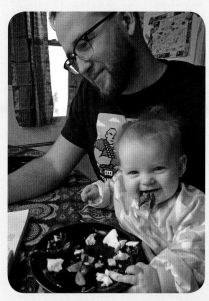
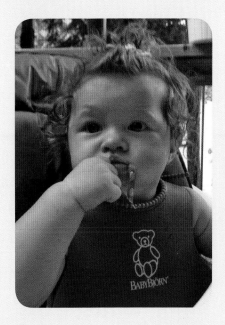
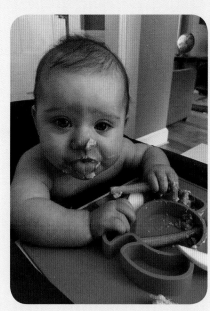

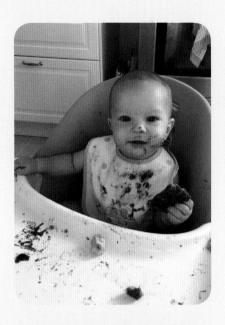

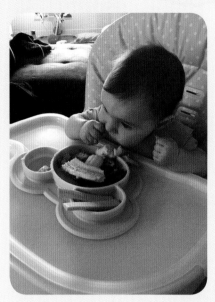

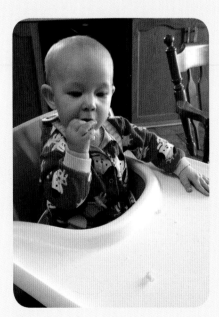

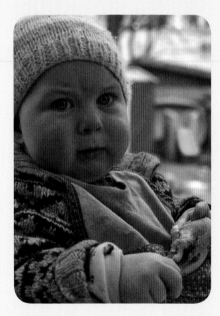

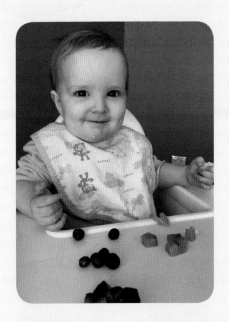

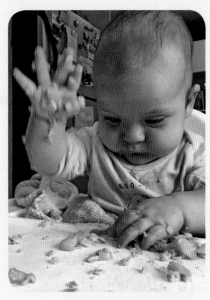

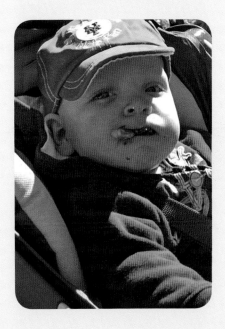

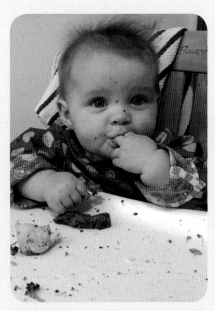

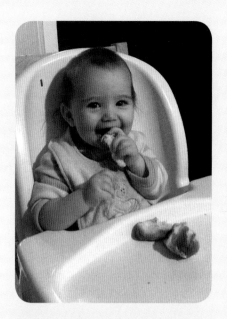 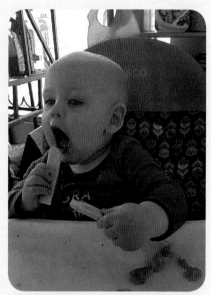

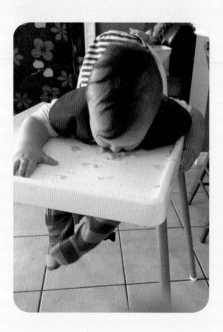 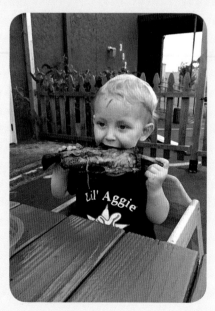

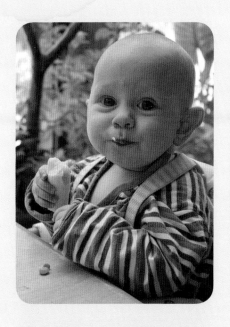
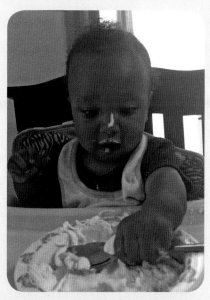
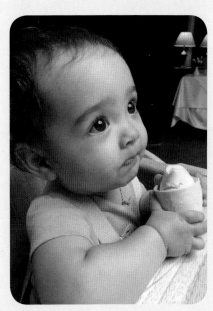
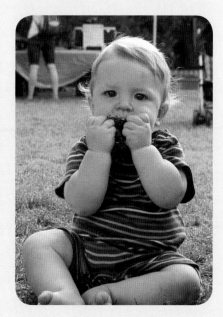

Bibliography

Abrams, E. M., and A. B. Becker. 2015. Food introduction and allergy prevention in infants. *CMAJ* 187 (17): 1297–301.

Ahmadizar, F., S. J. H. Viverberg, H. G. M. Arets, A. de Boer, J. E. Lang, J. Garssen, A. Kraneveld, and A. H. Maitland-van der Zee. 2017. Early-life antibiotic exposure increases the risk of developing allergic symptoms later in life: a meta-analysis. *Allergy* (November 6), doi: 10.1111/all.13332.

Apple, R. D. 1987. *Mothers and Medicine: A Social History of Infant Feeding 1890-1950.* Wisconsin: University of Wisconsin Press.

Batool, T., P. L. Reece, K. M. Morrison, S. A. Atkinson, S. S. Anand, K. K. Teo, J. A. Denburg, M. M. Cyr, and FAMILY Study Investigators. 2016. Prenatal and early-life predictors of atopy and allergic disease in Canadian children: results of the Family Atherosclerosis Monitoring In earLY life (FAMILY) Study. *J Dev Orig Health Dis* 7 (6): 665–71.

Birch, L.L., and A. E. Doub. 2014. Learning to eat: birth to age 2 y. *Am J Clin Nutr* 99 (3): 723S–8S.

Brown, A., S. Wyn-Jones, and H. Rowan. 2017. Baby-led weaning: the evidence to date. *Curr Nutr Rep* 6: 148–56.

Cameron, S. L., R. W. Taylor, and A. L. Heath. 2015. Development and pilot testing of Baby-Led Introduction to SolidS – a version of Baby-Led Weaning modified to address concerns about iron deficiency, growth faltering and choking. *BMC Pediatrics* 15: 99.

DeMuth, K., A. Stecenko, K. Sullivan, and A. Fitzpatrick. 2013. Relationship between treatment with antacid medication and the prevalence of food allergy in children. *Allergy Asthma Proc* 34 (3): 227–32.

Disantis, K. I., B. N. Collins, J. O. Fisher, and A. Davey. 2011. Do infants fed directly from the breast have improved appetite regulation and slower growth during early childhood compared with infants fed from a bottle?. *Int J Behav Nutr Phys Act* 8: 89.

Du Toit, G., Y. Katz, P. Sasieni, D. Mesher, S. J. Maleki, H. R. Fisher, A. T. Fox, et al. 2008. Early consumption of peanuts in infancy is associated with a low prevalence of peanut allergy. *J Allergy Clin Immunol* 122 (5): 984–91.

Greer, F. R., and R. D. Apple. 1991. Physicians, formula companies, and advertising: a historical perspective. *American Journal of Diseases of Children* 145 (3): 282–86.

Henderson, A.J., and S. O. Shaheen. 2013. Acetaminophen and asthma. *Pediatr Respir Rev* 14 (1): 9–15.

Huh, S. Y., S. L. Rifas-Shiman, E. M. Taveras, E. Oken, and M. W. Gillman. 2011. Timing of solid food introduction and risk of obesity in preschool-aged children. *Pediatrics* 127 (3): e544–e551.

Kc, A., N. Rana, M. Malqvist, L. Jarawka Ranneberg, K. Subedi, and O. Andersson. 2017. Effects of delayed umbilical cord clamping vs early clamping on anemia in infants at 8 and 12 months: a randomized clinical trial. *JAMA Pediatr* 171 (3): 264–70.

Kim, P., R. Feldman, L. C. Mayes, V. Eicher, N. Thompson, J. F. Leckman, and J. E. Swain. 2011. Breastfeeding, brain activation to own infant cry and maternal sensitivity. *J Child Psychol Psychiatry* 52 (8): 907–15.

Korpela, K., M.A. Zijlmans, M. Kuitunen, K. Kukkonen, E. Savilahti, A. Salonen, C. de Weerth, and W. M. de Vos. 2017. Childhood BMI in relation to microbiota in infancy and lifetime antibiotic use. *Microbiome* 5 (1): 26.

Li, R., S. B. Fein, and L. M. Grummer-Strawn. 2010. Do infants fed from bottles lack self-regulation of milk intake compared with directly breastfed infants? *Pediatrics* 125 (6): 1386–93.

Maier, A., C. Chabanet, B. Schaal, S. Issanchou, and P. Leathwood. 2007. Effects of repeated exposure on acceptance of initially disliked vegetables in 7-month old infants. *Food Quality and Preference* 18 (8): 1023–32.

Maier-Noth, A., B. Schaal, P. Leathwood, and S. Issanchou. 2016. The lasting influences of early food-related variety experience: a longitudinal study of vegetable acceptance from 5 months to 6 years in two populations. *PLoS* 11 (3), doi: 10.1371/journal.pone.0151356.

Martin, R. M, D. Gunnell, C. G. Owen, and G. D. Smith. 2005. Breast-feeding and childhood cancer: a systemic review with metaanalysis. *Int J Cancer* 117 (6): 1020–31.

Matheson, B. E., C. Camacho, C. B. Peterson, K. E. Rhee, S. A. Rydell, N. L. Zucker, and K. N. Boutelle. 2015. The relationship between parent feeding styles and general parenting with loss of control eating in treatment-seeking overweight and obese children. *Int J Eat Disord* 48 (7): 1047–55.

Morison, B. J., R. W. Taylor, J. J. Haszard, C. J. Schramm, L. Williams Erickson, L. J. Fangupo, E. A. Fleming, et al. 2016. How different are baby-led weaning and conventional complementary feeding? A cross-sectional study of infants aged 6–8 months. *BMJ Open*, doi: 10.1136/bmjopen-2015-010665.

Murthy, C. L., B. Bharti, P. Mathi, and A. Khadwal. 2015. Sleep habits and sleep problems in healthy preschoolers. *Indian J Pediatr* 82 (7): 606–11.

Newman, J., and T. Pitman. 2014. *Dr. Jack Newman's Guide to Breastfeeding*, revised edition. Toronto: Harper-Collins.

Radbill, S. X. 1981. Infant feeding through the ages. *Clinical Pediatrics* 20: 613–21.

Sbihi, H., R. W. Allen, A. Becker, J. R. Brook, P. Mandhane, J. A. Scott, M. R. Sears, et al. 2015. Perinatal exposure to traffic-related air pollution and atopy at 1 year of age in a multi-center Canadian birth cohort study. *Environ Health Perspect* 123 (9): 902–8.

Scott, F. J., D. B. Horton, R. Mamtani, K. Haynes, D. S. Goldberg, D. Y. Lee, and J. D. Lewis. 2016. Administration of antibiotics to children before age 2 years increases risk for childhood obesity. *Gastroenterology* 151 (1): 120–9.

Shim, J. E., J. Kim, R. A. Mathai, and STRONG Kids Research Team. 2011. Associations of infant feeding practices and picky eating behaviors of preschool children. *J Am Diet Assoc* 111 (9): 1363–8.

Shloim, N., L. R. Edelson, N. Martin, and M. M. Hetherington. 2015. Parenting styles, feeding styles, feeding practices and weight status in 4–12 year-old children: a systematic review of the literature. *Front Psychology* 6: 1849.

Smith, L. J., and M. Kroeger. 2009. *Impact of Birthing Practices on Breastfeeding*. New York: Jones and Bartlett Learning.

Taylor, R. W., S. M. Williams, L. J. Fangupo, B. J. Wheeler, B. J. Taylor, L. Daniels, E. A. Fleming, et al. 2017. Effect of a baby-led approach to complementary feeding on infant growth and overweight: a randomized clinical trial. *JAMA Pediatr* 171 (9): 838–46.

Wiessinger, D., D. West, and T. Pitman. 2010. *The Womanly Art of Breastfeeding*, 8th edition. New York: Ballantine Books.

Resources

Websites

www.rapleyweaning.com
www.llli.org
www.lllc.ca
You can also search Facebook for baby-led weaning groups in your area.

Books

*Baby-Led Weaning: The Essential Guide to Introducing Solid Foods —
and Helping Your Baby to Grow Up a Happy and Confident Eater*
by Gill Rapley and Tracey Murkett

The Parents' Guide to Baby-Led Weaning by Jennifer House

The Womanly Art of Breastfeeding (8th edition) by Diane Wiessinger,
Diana West and Teresa Pitman

Dr. Jack Newman's Guide to Breastfeeding (revised edition)
by Dr. Jack Newman and Teresa Pitman

Acknowledgments

I want to thank Lisa, Sascha and Isla for their help in telling the story of Isla's discovery of food. She still gets excited when her plate is set down in front of her!

Many thanks to the La Leche League Leaders who taught me about this approach to solid foods when my babies were small and all the parents I've worked with over the years who have found these ideas helpful.

Huge thanks to Steve and Julie at Firefly Books for all their work in bringing this book to life, Molly Roberts and Jennifer House for their expertise, Dreena Burton for sharing her experience as a vegan mom, Tania Craan for her lovely design, Reg Vertolli (and Quin) for their work behind the camera (Reg only made one baby cry!) and the many parents who shared their photos and stories with us.

And, of course, thank you Roberta Samec who started the ball rolling …

Picture Credits

Alamy Stock Photo:
  Jeff Morgan 06: 37
  M&N: 35
  Peter Horree: 31

Dreena Burton: 101

iStock Photo:
  Alija: 109
  FatCamera: 33
  lostinbids: 68
  Peopleimages: 158
  Weekend Images Inc.: 138

Reg Vertolli: 2, 8, 13, 14, 45, 64, 71, 77, 89,
  98, 105 (top), 121, 140, 177

Sascha von Nickisch-Rosenegk: 18, 20, 21, 23,
  24, 25, 47

Shutterstock:
  Africa Studio: 57, 73, 84, 127
  Akkalak Aiempradit: 61
  Alena Ozerova: 63
  Anna Kucherova: 108
  Atsushi Hirao: 174
  baibaz: 88, 165
  bergamont: 1 (nectarine), 3 (nectarine)
  Binh Thanh Bui: 86, 104
  BonNontawat: 96
  Brina L. Bunt: 29
  digieye: 114
  Dionisvera: 164
  espies: 52
  foxie: 3 (banner)
  Garsya: 81
  Iurii Kachkovskyi: 79
  Kateryna Bibro: 1 (broccoli), 105 (bottom)
  komokvm: 87, 107
  Kovaleva_Ka: 131
  Lopolo: 117
  maramorosz: 112
  Marko Poplasen: 72

Maryna Pleshkun: 124
Mcimage: 41, 78
Moving Moment: 154
Myibean: 170
optimarc: 103
pixelheadphoto digitalskillet: 49
Romrodphoto: 59
schankz: 1 (hand)
Skylines: 118
Suslik1983: 111
Syda Productions: 93
timquo: 163
ValeStock: 28
Viktar Malyshchyts: 132
zlikovec: 133
ZouZou: 55

Stocksy United:
  Bo Bo: 56
  Inuk Studio: 70
  Kelly Knox: 26
  Kristen Curette Hines: 129
  Lauren Naefe: 74
  Photographer Christian B: 94
  Sean Locke: 91
  Tara Romasanta: 130

Front Cover:
Shutterstock:
  bergamont (nectarine); foxie (banner);
  Kateryna Bibro (broccoli); schankz (hand)

Back Cover: Reg Vertolli

We would like to thank all the parents who
submitted photos for the Appendix: Baby-Led
Weaning in Practice.

Index